MICROBIOLOGY CLASS NOTES

THE BIG PICTURE

TRAMAR F. MURDOCK, MD

These notes are aimed in organizing and providing general principles of Microbiology to my students.

authorHOUSE®

AuthorHouse™
1663 Liberty Drive
Bloomington, IN 47403
www.authorhouse.com
Phone: 1 (800) 839-8640

Published by AuthorHouse   08/07/2015

ISBN: 978-1-5049-2405-4 (sc)
ISBN: 978-1-5049-2404-7 (e)

Library of Congress Control Number: 2015911947

Print information available on the last page.

Any people depicted in stock imagery provided by Thinkstock are models, and such images are being used for illustrative purposes only. Certain stock imagery © Thinkstock.

This book is printed on acid-free paper.

Contents

ACKNOWLEDGEMENTS AND SPECIAL THANKS TO

Garry S. Jennings, MD
QOL Pain Management, Inc.
Friend, Husband, and Supporter

Dr. Elmer Pfefferkorn
Dartmouth Medical School
Microbiology
Mentor

Vincent Memoli, MD
Dartmouth Medical School
Pathology
Friend and Mentor

BIBLIOGRAPHY

1. Gladwin M, Trattler B. <u>Clinical Microbiology Made Ridiculously Simple</u>; 2nd edition. MediMaster, Inc., Miami, 1997.
2. Tortora j, Funke B, Case C, et al. <u>Microbiology: An Introduction</u>; 11th edition. Pearson Education, Inc., publishing as Benjamin Cummings, San Francisco, CA, 2005.

MICROBIOLOGY

INTRODUCTION/BRIEF HISTORY

A. Microbiology
- The study of minute living things (**microorganisms**) which live around us and /or inside us
- Usually too small to be seen by the unaided eye

B. What is an Organism
- A living thing (**animal, plant, single cell**)
- "Takes in" and "breaks down" food for energy and nutrients; excretes undigested food as waste
- Reproduce

C. Friendly Microorganisms
- Majority of **Microorganisms** help **maintain balance** of living organisms and chemicals in the environment
  - **Flora organisms** in the intestines help **digest food; help form Vitamins (B, K)**
- Used in producing **foods, drugs, chemicals, alcohol, enzymes**

D. Unfriendly Microorganisms
- **Pathogenic** microbes: produce **disease**
- Cause **Infection(s)**: invasion of disease causing microorganisms
  - *Entameoba histolytica* (causes **Traveler's diarrhea**)
  - *Mycobacterium tuberculosis* (causes **TB**)

E. Major Groups
- **Bacteria** (singular: **bacterium**)
  - **Bacteriology:** study of **Bacteria**
  - **Prokaryotic organisms** (simple **single-celled/unicellular** organisms)
  - Genetic material **not enclosed** in a **nuclear membrane**
  - Reproduce by **binary fissure** (divide into 2 equal parts)
  - Most use organic chemicals for nutrition
  - Some manufacture food by **photosynthesis**
  - Some have **flagella** (motility)
  - Cell wall composed of **peptidoglycan**
  - Several shapes and forms
- **Archaea**
  - **Prokaryotic cells**
  - Cell wall **lacks** peptidoglycan
  - Found in **extreme environments**
  - Three groups: **methanogens** (produce methane), **halophiles** (salt loving), **extreme thermophiles** (heat)
- **Viruses** (singular: **virus**)
  - **Virology:** study **of viruses**
  - **Submicroscopic, acellular, parasitic** entities made up of a **core of DNA or RNA,** surrounded by a **protein coat**
  - **Reproduce** only by using the **"Host" cellular machinery**

- **Fungi (singular: fungus)**
  - o **Mycology:** study of **Fungi**
  - o **Eukaryotic** (cells have a <u>**distinct nucleus**</u> containing **DNA** surrounded by a **nuclear membrane**)
  - o Unicellular or multicellular
  - o **Cell wall** composed of substance called **chitin**
  - o **Do not** carry out **photosynthesis**
  - o **Yeast, molds, mushrooms**
- **Algae (singular: alga)**
  - o **Phycology:** study of **Algae**
  - o **Eukaryotic Photosynthetic organisms**
  - o **Cell wall** of many composed of **cellulose**
  - o Abundant in freshwater, saltwater, soil, and associated with plants
  - o Do not generally require organic compounds from the environment
  - o Produce **oxygen and carbohydrates** used by other organisms
- **Protozoa (singular:protozoan)**
  - o **Protozoology:** study of **Protozoa**
  - o Animal-like **unicellular eukaryotic organisms**
  - o Found in **aquatic and terrestrial places**
  - o Some **photosynthetic**
  - o Move by **pseudopods, flagella, or cilia**
  - o Ingest or absorb organic compounds
- **Parasites**
  - o **Parasitology:** study of **parasites**
  - o Lives at the expense of another organism or host
  - o Worms (**helminths**), insects, certain bacteria, viruses

F. Naming and Classification of Microorganisms
- **Naming: Carl Linnaeus (1735)**
  - o Used **Two Names** (Latin)
    - ■ 1st name: **Genus** (plural **genera**); always **CAPITALIZED**
    - ■ 2nd name: **Specific epithet** (species name); **not capitalized**
    - ■ Both names <u>**underlined**</u> or *italicized*

Staphylococcus aureus

clustered   circular   golden

Escherichia coli

Theodor Escherich   lives in colon

- **Classification: Carl Woese (1978)**
  - o Based on **molecular and cellular characteristics**
  - o **Three** Domains
    - ■ **Bacteria:** peptidoglycan cell walls
    - ■ **Archaea:** <u>lack</u> peptidoglycan in cell wall (if cell wall present)
    - ■ **Eukarya:Organisms from the following kingdoms**
      - ✓ **Protists:** algae, protozoa, slime molds
      - ✓ **Fungi:** unicellular yeasts, multicellular molds, mushrooms

    ✓ **Plants:** moss, conifers, ferns, flowering plants
    ✓ **Animals:** insects, sponges, worms, vertebrates

G. First Observations

- **Zacharias Janssen (1590)**
  - Believed to have developed first Compound Microscope (3 tubes)
- **Robert Hooke (1665)**
  - Viewed **slices of cork (non living)** and saw "little boxes" which he called **"cells"**
  - Lead to development of **"Cell Theory"**
- **Antoni Van Leeuwenhoek (1673)**
  - Improved Hooke's microscope
  - First person to view **"a living"** organism (**Animalcules**)

H. Spontaneous versus Non-Spontaneous Generation

- **Spontaneous Generation**
  - **Originally** thought some **living organisms** arouse from <u>**non-living matter**</u>
- **Non-Spontaneous Generation**
  - **Francesco Redi (1668)**
    - Proved organisms did not spontaneously appear
    - Experiment with jars containing decayed meat
  - **John Needham (1745)**
    - Microbes **arise** from **heated nutrient** fluids (chicken and corn broth), after covered and cooled
  - **Lazzaro Spallanzani (1765)**
    - Nutrient fluids heated **after** being covered did not grow microbes; **microbes in air entered**

I. Theory of Biogenesis

- **Rudolf Virchow (1858)**
  - **Living** cells come from **preexisting living** cells
- **Louis Pasteur (1861)**
  - **Microorganisms** are present in the **air, nonliving matter, and contaminate sterile things**
    - **Aseptic technique**

J. Fermentation and Pasteurization

- Methods used to **prevent spoilage**
  - **Pasteurization:** a technique which **kills most bacteria** that cause spoilage **by heating to a certain temperature**
  - **Fermentation:** anaerobic (without oxygen) **cellular process** in which organic foods are converted into simpler compounds, and chemical energy is produced; occurs in certain bacteria, yeast
    - Converts sugar to acids, gases, and/or alcohol, in the absence of air

K. Germ Theory of Disease

- A Contagion (**microorganism**) can cause a **disease**
  - **Agostino Bassi (1835):** identified a fungus causing silkworm disease
  - **Louis Pasteur (1865):** protozoan afflicting silkworm moths causing disease
  - **Joseph Lister (1867):** used carbonic acid (phenol) for surgical wounds
- **Robert Koch (1876)**
  - **Koch's postulates**
  - Proved **specific microorganisms** caused **specific diseases**
    - *Bacillus anthracis* causes the disease **Anthrax**

L. Vaccination
- **Edward Jenner (1796)**
  - o Inoculated healthy person with tiny amount of disease causing organisms
  - o **Inoculation** with **cowpox** provided **humans immunity** to **smallpox**
  - o Protection from a disease provided by vaccination **called <u>immunity</u>**
- **Vaccines produced from:** living avirulent microbes, killed pathogens, parts of virulent microbes, and recombinant DNA techniques

M. Birth of Modern Chemotherapy
- **Chemotherapy**
  - o **Treatment** of infectious (microbes) and noninfectious (cancers) diseases **using chemical substances**
  - o **"Drug"** that will **kill pathogen without harming the infected host**
    - ■ **Synthetic drugs:** prepared from chemicals in the lab
      - ✓ **Paul Ehrlich (1890)**
      - ✓ <u>Salvarsan</u> **(arsenic derivative)** effective against **syphilis**
      - ✓ Quinine-malaria
      - ✓ Sulfonamides (sulfa drug)-bacterial infections
    - ■ **Antibiotics**-chemicals produced naturally by bacteria or fungi
      - ❖ **Alexander Flemming**
- **Problems with Synthetic Drugs and Antibiotics**
  - o **Toxicity**
  - o **New Strains** emerging

N. Genomics
- The study of an organisms genes to help classify bacteria, fungi, protozoan
- **Recombinant DNA Technology**
  - o **Technique** using **fragments of DNA** (human/animal) that **code for certain proteins** (genes) and **attach these "genes" to bacterial DNA**
  - o The **recombinant DNA is inserted into bacteria** (or other microbes); used to **make large quantities** of the desired protein

O. Microbes and Human Welfare
- The **majority** of microbes **benefit** humans, animals, plants
  - o **Recycling:** microbes recycle elements between soil and the atmosphere
    - ■ Microbial Ecology
  - o **Sewage Treatment:** recycle water
  - o **Bioremediation:** microbes used to clean up pollutants and toxic waste
  - o **Insect Pest Control:** important for agricultural
  - o **Biotechnology and Recombinant DNA Technology:** commercial use of microbes to produce common foods and chemicals
    - ■ **Gene Therapy:** inserting a missing gene or replacing defective one

P. Microbes and Human Disease
- **Normal Microbiota**
  - o Outside and inside the Body
  - o **Normal microbiota (flora), DO NOT HARM US!**
- **Biofilms**
  - o Complex **aggregate** of microbes
  - o Beneficial (protective layer, food) or harmful (cause infections, clog pipes)

- **Infectious Disease**
  - o **Pathogens invade host** causing disease
- **Emerging Infectious Diseases (EIDs)**
  - o Certain infectious diseases are **reemerging** and **increasing**
  - o Due to evolutionary changes
    - ■ **H1N1 influenza (flu)**
    - ■ **Avian influenza (H5N1)**or **bird flu**
    - ■ **Methicillin-resistant** *Staphylococcus aureus* **(MRSA)**
    - ■ **Vancomycin-resistant** *Staphylococcus aureus* **(VRSA)**
- **Emerging Infectious Diseases (EIDs)**
  - o **West Nile encephalitis (WNE)**
  - o **Bovine spongioform encephalopathy (BSE** or **mad cow disease)**
  - o **Ebola hemorrhagic fever (EHF)**
  - o **Human immunodeficiency virus (HIV)**

MICROBIOLOGY

CHEMICAL PRINCIPLES/ELEMENTS OF MICROBIOLOGY

A. Microorganisms are made up of Chemicals
- **An organism is** also known as **"A Chemical Processing Plant"**
- Take **"things"**, brake them down, rearrange these "things" into forms which **provide nutrients and energy**
- **Chemistry** is the science of the interactions between **atoms and molecules**

B. Chemical Elements and the Atom
- All **matter** (rock, air, **living organisms**) is made up of **Atoms**

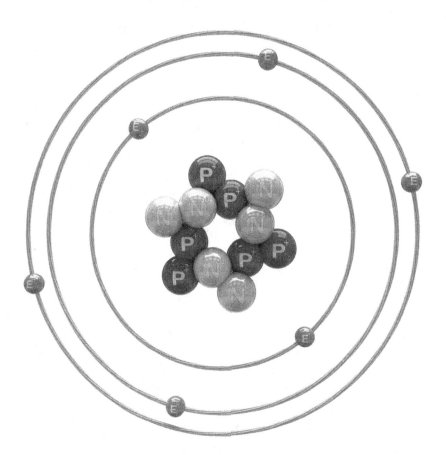

- **Atom** is the **smallest unit** of a **chemical element**
- Consist of
  - **Nucleus:** central, usually stable; consists of **proton (+) and neutron (o)**
  - **Shell:** outer, surrounds nucleus; consist of **electrons (-)** moving around nucleus; region of different energy levels
- **Atoms** listed by their **atomic number : # protons** in nucleus
- **Atomic weight: total # of protons and neutrons**

- **Chemical Element (s)**
  - o **A pure chemical substance** consisting of a **single atom distinguished by its atomic number**
    - Example : **Carbon (C)**
  - o **Isotopes:** atoms with **different #'s** of **neutrons,** but **same # protons** in the **nucleus**
    - Cause **difference in atomic weights**
    - Example: **Oxygen (O)**; has three isotopes
- **Electronic Configurations**
  - o Consists of electrons arranged around the nucleus in electron shells
  - o Each shell holds a maximum # of electrons
  - o Filled shells: **Stable, inert**
  - o Outer electron shell partially filled: **Unstable, reacts**

C. Chemical Reaction (s)

- Process of **bonding together atoms** and **separating atoms already bonded**
- Occurs by **gaining, losing, or sharing** electrons from outer shell
- **Rearranging, combining, separating elements**
- Requires **energy**
- **Chemical reactions**
  - o **Endergonic:** absorbs more energy that expels
  - o **Exergonic:** expels (releases) more energy than absorbed
- **Three (3) Types of Chemical Reactions**
  - o **Synthesis:** 2 or more atoms, ions, molecules **bind together** forming a **larger molecule**
    - **Anabolic/Anabolism**
      $A + B \rightarrow AB$
  - o **Decomposition: breaks down** into **smaller parts**
    - **Catabolic/Catabolism**
      $AB \rightarrow A + B$
  - o **Exchange/Displacement**
    - **Anabolic and Catabolic**
      $AB + C \rightarrow AC + B$
      $AB + CD \rightarrow AC + BD$

D. Reversibility of Chemical Reactions

- Occur in **either direction**
  - o $A + B \leftrightarrow AB$
    - Due to reactants and products being unstable
    - Special conditions

E. Chemical Bond (s)

- Causes stabilization
  - o **Diatomic:** 2 atoms of the same element bond (H-H= H_2)
  - o **Compound:** 2 atoms of different chemical elements bind (H-O-H=H_2O)
- **Chemical Bonds** can be:
  - o **Ionic:** <u>attraction</u> between ions of **opposite charge**
    - Ex. NaCl
  - o **Covalent:** atoms <u>share</u> one or > pairs of electrons; <u>**strong bonds**</u>
    - Ex. H_2
  - o **Hydrogen :**<u>**weak temporary bond**</u>; a hydrogen atom bonded to one oxygen or nitrogen atom is attracted to another oxygen or nitrogen atom; **bridge between different molecules**
    - Ex. H_2O

- **Molecular Weight and Moles**
  - o **Molecular weight:** the sum of the atomic weighs of all its atoms
  - o **Mole:** is the molecular weight expressed in **grams**

F. Chemical Compounds
- Divided into Groups
  - o **Inorganic: lack carbon (C) molecule; <u>ionic bonds</u> significant**
  - o **Organic: contains carbon and hydrogen; <u>covalent bonds</u> significant**
- **Inorganic Compounds**
  - o **Water**
    - ▪ **Most important** and **most abundant**
    - ▪ Required for life: growth, repair, reproduction
    - ▪ A **polar molecule**
- **Inorganic Compounds**
  - o **Acids**
    - ▪ Dissociates into 1 or > Hydrogen ions (H^+) and 1 or > negative ions (anions); a proton donor
  - o **Bases**
    - ▪ Dissociates into 1 or > positive ions (cations) plus 1 or > negative OH^- ions: an electron acceptor
  - o **Salts**
    - ▪ Dissociates into 1 or > cations ($^+$) and anions($^-$) ions, in H_2O
    - ▪ The ($^+$) or ($^-$) ions are neither H^+ or OH^-

  - o **Acid-Base Balance: pH Concept**
    - ▪ **The pH scale:** measures **acidity or alkalinity** of a substance
      - ✓ pH 7: neutral
      - ✓ pH < 7: acid
      - ✓ pH >7: base
    - ▪ **Buffer:** either releases (H^+) or binds (H^+) **to stabilize pH**
- **Organic Compounds**
  - o Contain **carbon and hydrogen elements**
  - o Carbon plays vital role in living things
  - o Large organic compounds called **polymers**
  - o **Polymers:** made up of small molecules **(monomers)**
  - o Large organic compound called **a macromolecule (aka polymer)**
  - o **Four Groups of Organic Molecules**
    - ▪ <u>**Carbohydrates**</u>
      - ✓ Include sugar, starches, cellulose, glycogen
      - ✓ Made up of **carbon, hydrogen, oxygen atoms**
      - ✓ <u>**Monosaccharides**</u>
        - ❖ Simple sugars
        - ❖ **Glucose, fructose, galactose, D (deoxyribose)NA, R (ribose)NA**
      - ✓ <u>**Disaccharides**</u>
        - ❖ Two monosaccharides bond
        - ❖ **Sucrose:**
        - ❖ **Lactose:**
        - ❖ **Maltose:**
      - ✓ <u>**Polysaccharides**</u>
        - ❖ Tens or hundreds of monosaccharides bond
        - ❖ **Glycogen, starch, cellulose, chitin, dextran**

- <u>**Lipids**</u>
  - ✓ **Fats** which provide **protection, insulation, energy**
  - ✓ Important to **cell membranes**
  - ✓ <u>**Simple Lipids**</u>
    - ❖ **Triglycerides**
      -Contain glycerol and fatty acids; mostly insoluble
      -Important in **plasma membrane**
      -**Protect and insulate body**
      -Saturated versus Unsaturated
  - ✓ <u>**Complex Lipids**</u>
    - ❖ **Phospholipids**
      *Contain glycerol, 2 fatty acids, phosphate group
      *Build **cell membrane**
    - ❖ **Glycolipids**
      *Lipid with carbohydrates attached
  - ✓ <u>**Steroids**</u>
    - ❖ **Cholesterol and some hormones**
      *Structurally different from lipids
      *Important component of plasma membrane

- <u>**Proteins**</u>
  - ✓ Contain carbon, hydrogen, oxygen, nitrogen (some sulphur)
  - ✓ Hundreds of different proteins found in a cell
  - ✓ Some are antibodies that kill bacteria, transporters, enzymes, toxins
  - ✓ Make up cell structures, cytoplasmic organelles, movement, hormones
  - ✓ Made up of **amino acids** which are **bonded together** by **peptide bonds**
  - ✓ <u>**Four Structural Levels**</u>
    - ❖ **Primary:** aa's linked to form a polypeptide chain
    - ❖ **Secondary:** localized, repetitious twisting or folding of the polypeptide chain; helix or pleated sheets
    - ❖ **Tertiary:** three-dimensional folding of the structure
    - ❖ **Quaternary:** several polypeptide chains that make up a protein
  - ✓ **Have many roles in a living organism**
  - ✓ Muscle contraction
  - ✓ Hemoglobin
  - ✓ Motility

- <u>**Nucleic acids**</u>
  - ✓ First discovered in the nuclei of cells
  - ✓ Made up of **nucleotides (**consisting of a base, sugar, phosphate group)
  - ✓ <u>**2 Types**</u>
    - ❖ **DNA**
      * <u>**Deoxyribose**</u>
      *Double stranded (ds); forms a double helix; organized into segments (gene)
      *Bases: A, G, C, <u>**T**</u>
      *Stores genetic information
    - ❖ **RNA**
      *<u>**Ribose**</u>
      *Single stranded (ss)
      *Bases: A, G, C, <u>**U**</u>
      *Function in protein synthesis

G. Adenosine Triphosphate (ATP) Molecules
- **Principle energy-carrying molecule**
- Stores and supplies energy
- High energy molecule
- Supplies energy for:
  - Examples
    - Flagella
    - Moving chromosomes
    - Transports substances in and out of the plasma membrane
- **Synthesized from ADP and P**
- **Releases energy in the form of ADP and P**

MICROBIOLOGY

OBSERVING MICROORGANISMS

A. Metric System
- Used to **measure** microorganisms
- **Standard unit of length: the meter (m)**

-
Metric Unit	Prefix	Metric Equivalent
o 1 Kilometer (km)	kilo = 1000	1000m = 10^3 m
o 1 Meter (m)		**STANDARD UNIT**
o 1 Decimeter (dm)	deci =1/10	0.1m = 10^{-1} m
o 1 Centimeter (cm)	centi = 1/100	0.01 m = 10^{-2} m
o 1 Millimeter (mm)	milli = 1/1,000	0.001m = 10^{-3} m
o 1 Micrometer (μm)	micro = 1/1,000,000	0.000001m = 10^{-6} m
o 1 Nanometer (nm)	nano = 1/1,000,000,000	0.000000001m = 10^{-9} m
o 1Picometer (pm)	pico = 1/1,000,000,000,000	0.000000000001m=10^{-12} m

B. Microscopy: The Instruments
- **Microscopes** are devices that **enlarge objects** using a process called magnification
- **Simplest microscope is a "magnifying glass"**

C. Light Microscopy
- Uses **visible light** to examine specimens
- **Simple:** consist of **a single lens**
- **Compound:** consists of **multiple lenses (ocular and objective)**
  - o Parts of a **compound light microscope**
    - ■ **Frame**
      - ✓ Arm:
      - ✓ Base:
      - ✓ Body:
    - ■ **Stage**
      - ✓ Supports the microscopic slide; may have a clamping device
    - ■ **Illuminator**
      - ✓ Light source
    - ■ **Condenser**
      - ✓ Condenses, collects, and directs light from light source to slide
    - ■ **Diaphragm**
      - ✓ Adjust amount of light that reaches the specimen
    - ■ **Objectives**
      - ✓ Two or more lenses
      - ✓ Closest to specimen; attached to nose piece (10X, 45X, 100X-oil)
    - ■ **Ocular**
      - ✓ Eye piece; specimen magnified again
    - ■ **Focusing knobs**

- ✓ Brings objects into focus
  - ❖ **Coarse adjustment**
  - ❖ **Fine adjustment**
- **Total Magnification**
  - o Used to calculate the total magnification of a specimen
  - o <u>**Multiply**</u> the **objective lens** power (Example: 10X, 45X, 100X) **by the ocular lens power (factor of 10)**
- **Resolution**
  - o Also called **resolving power**
  - o **The ability of the lenses to distinguish fine detail and structure**
  - o The ability of the lenses to distinguish between two points at specified distance apart
  - o Minimum distance one can see two adjacent objects
- **Refractive Index**
  - o A **measure** of the **light-bending** ability **of the medium**
  - o Changed by **staining**
  - o **Refracted**
  - o **Oil immersion**

D. Microscopy

- **Bright field**
  - o Stained specimens; brightly illuminated
- **Darkfield**
  - o Examines **live organisms** that are invisible in ordinary light, cannot be stained, or distorted by staining
  - o Uses a **condenser** containing an **opaque disc** which blocks light **(light reflected away)**
  - o Specimen is **"light" against a dark background**
  - o *Treponema palladium* (syphilis)
- **Phase-Contrast Microscopy**
  - o Examine **detailed internal structures** in <u>**unstained living microorganisms**</u>
  - o Special **diaphragm**
- **Differential Interference Contrast (DIC)**
  - o Uses **two beams of light separated <u>by prisms</u>**
  - o **Specimen** appears **colored due to prism effect** (3D images)
- **Fluorescence Microscopy**
  - o Uses **UV light** to illuminate specimens
  - o Fluorescent dyes **called fluorchromes used**
  - o **Stains microbes bright apple green, or bright yellow**
  - o *Mycobacterium tuberculosis* (tuberculosis)
  - o For immunofluorescence techniques
- **Confocal Microscopy**
  - o Uses **fluorochromes**; uses a **pinhole aperature**
  - o Illuminated with short wavelength light
  - o Used with **computers to** produces two and three-dimensional images; see inside cell
  - o Uses lasers
- **Two-Photon Microscopy (TPM)**
  - o **Living specimen** dyed with fluorescent dye
  - o Uses **long-wave (red) light** therefore two photons needed
  - o Can track **"cell activity"** in real time
- **Scanning Acoustic Microscopy (SAM)**
  - o Uses a **sound wave that** travels **through the specimen to examine living cells**

- o Study **living cells attached to another surface (biofilms)**
- ● **Electron Microscopy**
  - o Examines **viruses and internal structures of microorganisms (<0.2 μm)**
  - o Uses **beams of electrons** on the specimen (in a vacuum)
  - o Instead of **glass lens,** uses **electromagnetic lenses**
  - o Microscopic photographs called **micrographs**
  - o <u>**Two Types**</u>
    - ■ Transmission Electron Microscope **(TEM)**
      - ✓ Structures **smaller than 0.2 μm** can be **examined**
      - ✓ Examine ultra thin section of specimen
      - ✓ **Image produced is two-dimensional**
      - ✓ Examine **viruses or internal structures**
    - ■ Scanning Electron Microscope **(SEM)**
      - ✓ **Image produced is three-dimensional**
      - ✓ Studies **surface features of cells and viruses**
- ● **Scanned-Probe Microscopy**
  - o Uses **thin metal probe** which **scans a specimen**
  - o Produces bumps and depressions of the atoms on the surface of the specimen
  - o Provides **detailed views of molecules inside cells**
  - o <u>**Two Types**</u>
    - ■ Scanning Tunneling Microscopy **(STM)**
      - ✓ Provide **detailed views of molecules such as DNA**
    - ■ Atomic Force Microscopy **(AFM)**
      - ✓ Uses **metal-and-diamond probe** on specimen
      - ✓ Provides **images of molecular processes and biological molecules**

E. Preparing Specimens for Light Microscopy
- ● When viewed most microorganisms appear **"colorless"**
- ● **Preparations include the following**
  - o **Fixed (or fixation)**
    - ■ **Attaches** specimen to the slide
    - ■ **Kills the microorganisms** and **preserves various parts with minimal distortion**
    - ■ Can be alcohol, heat, formalin
  - o **Wet mount**
    - ■ **Live specimen** placed on a **concave or plain slide**
  - o **Smear**
    - ■ **Preparation process** where a **thin layer of material** (containing the **specimen**) is spread on a slide; air dried or passed through a flame
  - o **Stains (Staining)**
    - ■ Giving **something that is colorless "color";** use **dyes**
    - ■ **Salts** made up of **positive ion and negative ion**
    - ■ **Positive or negative ion** can be colored; known as a **chromophore**
    - ■ The color of **basic dyes is in the positive ion**
      - ✓ **Basic dyes:** crystal violet, ethylene blue, safranin, malachite green
    - ■ The color of **acidic dyes is in the negative ion**
      - ✓ **Acidic dyes:** eosin, acid fuchsin, nigrosin
    - ■ Bacteria are slightly negatively charged at pH 7; Colored positive charge ion in a basic dye will be attracted to the negatively charged bacterial cell
    - ■ **Negative staining: prepare "colorless" specimens against a "colored" background**

F. Types of Stains
- **Simple Stains**
  - o **Alcohol or aqueous solution** made up of a <u>single</u> **basic dye**
  - o Shows **shapes** of cells; some **structures within a cell**
  - o **Mordants** (intensify the stain: flagella)
  - o Examples: methylene blue, carbofuchsin, CV, safranin
- **Differential Stains**
  - o Consists of **two or more dyes**
  - o Used to **identify different kinds of bacteria**
  - o <u>**Two most commonly used differential stains**</u>
    - ■ <u>**Gram Stain**</u> (**Hans Christian Gram 1884**)
      - ✓ Classifies bacteria : **Gram (+) or Gram (-)**
      - ✓ **Steps**
        - ❖ Heat-fixed smear covered with a **purple dye (Crystal Violet:CV)**
        - ❖ **Crystal Violet (CV) a <u>Primary stain</u>; colors all cells**
        - ❖ Rinse
        - ❖ **Cover with Mordant (Iodine)**
        - ❖ Rinse: **Gram (+) and Gram (-) are blue/purple**
        - ❖ **Decolorize:** usually alcohol or acetone-alcohol solution; **removes blue/ purple from cells of one species but not other**
        - ❖ Rinse
        - ❖ <u>**Safranin**</u>: **(red dye); Counterstain**
        - ❖ Wash, blot, **examine**
      - ✓ **Gram (+) positive: Blue**
      - ✓ **Gram (-) negative: Red**
    - ■ <u>**Acid Fast Stain**</u>
      - ✓ **Carbolfuchsin: red dye; attaches to "waxy" material in cell walls** of bacteria such as *Mycobacterium tuberculosis (TB), Mycobacterium leprae(leprosy), Norcardia*
      - ✓ **Steps**
        - ❖ **Carbolfuchsin**
        - ❖ Heat (penetration, retention of dye)
        - ❖ Cooled, Rinse
        - ❖ **Decolorize:** acid-alcohol
        - ❖ Rinse
        - ❖ **Conterstain: Methylene blue**
- **Special Stains/Structural Stains**
  - o Used to **color and isolate specific parts** of microorganisms
    - ■ **Negative Staining**
      - ✓ For **capsules;** appear as halos; *(Klebsiella pneumoniae)*
    - ■ **Endospore (spore) Staining**
      - ✓ For **resistant, dormant structures (endospores)** formed within a cell to protect the bacterium from adverse environmental conditions. *(Bacillus cereus)*
    - ■ **Flagella Staining**
      - ✓ Demonstrate **flagella** (structures of locomotion)

MICROBIOLOGY

ANATOMY OF PROKARYOTIC AND EUKARYOTIC CELLS

A. Prokaryotic and Eukaryotic cells
- **Chemically similar** (nucleic acids, proteins, lipids, carbohydrates)
- Use **same chemical reactions** to metabolize foods, build proteins, store energy
- **Distinguished by cell walls, membranes, absence and/or presence of organelles**

B. Prokaryotic Cells
- Include **Bacteria and Archaea**
- **Lacks membrane-bound nucleus and organelles**
- Nuclear structure called "**Nucleoid**"; <u>usually</u> **single circular double stranded (ds) DNA**
- **DNA** not associated with **histones**
- **Cell wall** almost always contain **peptidoglycan**
- Usually **divide by binary fission**

C. Bacteria Sizes and Shapes
- **Many sizes and several shapes;** hereditary
  - **Monomorphic:** single shape, most bacteria
  - **Pleomorphic:** many shapes
- **Coccus** (plural:**cocci**)
  - **Spherical, round, oval**
    - **Diplococci:**
    - **Streptococci:**
    - **Tetrad:**
    - **Sarcinae:**
    - **Staphylococci:**
- **Bacillus** (plural: **bacilli**)
  - **Rod shaped**
    - **Diplobacilli:**
    - **Streptobacilli:**
    - **Coccobacilli:**
- **Spiral**
  - **One or > twists**
    - **Vibrio:**
    - **Spirilla:**
    - **Spirochetes:**
- **Other Shapes**
  - Star-shaped:
  - Rectangular-shaped:
  - Triangular-shaped:

D. Structures External Prokaryotic Cell Wall
- **Glycocalyx**
  - Made inside cell and secreted to surface

o **Sticky, sugary, gelatinous** material; made **of polysaccharides, polypeptides or both**
o **Protection; virulence; adhesion**
o **Capsule**: organized; firmly attached to cell wall
o **Slime layer**: unorganized; loosely attached to cell wall
o **Extracellular polymeric substance (EPS)**: helps cell attach to target environment and to each other

D. Structures External Prokaryotic Cell Wall
● **Flagella (singular: flagellum)**
  o **Long filamentous appendages; motility**
    ■ *Swim or Run→Tumbles→Swim or Run*
  o Semirigid; moves by **rotating**(clockwise or counterclockwise) from basal body
  o Propel organism **away (repellent)** or **toward (attractant)** particular stimuli: called **Taxis**
    ■ **Photo taxis:**
    ■ **Chemo taxis:**
  o Exist in several forms
    ■ **Atrichous: absent; without**
    ■ **Peritrichous: surrounds** entire cell
    ■ **Polar: at one or both poles**
      ✓ **Monotrichous: single** flagellum **at one pole**
      ✓ **Amphitrichous: single** flagellum **at both poles**
      ✓ **Lophotrichous: 2 or >** flagella **(tuft) at one or both poles**
      ✓ **Cephalotrichous:**
    ■ **Endoflagella (aka Axial Filaments)**
      ✓ **Bundles of fibrils** arising from ends of the cell beneath an outer sheath; **tightly wrapped** around the cell; anchored at one end
      ✓ **Propels** the microbe in a **spiral motion**
  o **Made up of Three Basic Parts**
    ■ **Filament: long outer region;** contains protein **flagellin**
    ■ **Hook:** filament attached
    ■ **Basal body: anchors flagella to cell wall and plasma membrane**
  o **Flagellar protein (H antigen):** used to distinguish among **serovars** or variations within a species of **gram (-) bacteria**
● **Fimbriae and Pili**
  o **Sticky, "bristle-like" projections;** shorter, straighter, thinner than flagella
  o Made of the protein **pilin**
    ■ **Fimbriae (singular: fimbria)**
      ✓ Few to hundred/cell
      ✓ Used mostly to **adhere to surfaces** (including other cells)
      ✓ Involved in forming **biofilms** and other aggregates on surfaces
    ■ **Pili (singular: pilus)**
      ✓ Longer than fimbria; one to two/cell
      ✓ Used for **motility**
        ❖ Twitching:
        ❖ Gliding:
      ✓ **Transfer DNA from** one cell to another
        ❖ Called **conjugation (sex) pili**

E. The Cell Wall
- Outside the **plasma membrane: porous; semi-rigid**
- Gives **cell shape and support**
- **Protection**
- **Resist pressures to prevent rupturing**
- Composed of **Peptidoglycan (aka murein)**
- **Peptidoglycan** made up of **a repeating <u>disaccharide</u> attached by <u>polypeptides</u>;** forms a lattice that surrounds entire cell
- **Disaccharides** made up of monosaccharides **called NAG and NAM**
- Penicillin: works on cell wall→lysis→loss of cytoplasmic contents
- **Gram Positive (+) Cell Walls**
  - o **Many layers of Peptidoglycan (PG)**
  - o **Contain Techoic Acids (alcohol and phosphate)**
    - ■ **Negatively (-) charged; may regulate positive (+) ions moving in and out of cell**
    - ■ Prevents wall breakdown and cell lyses
    - ■ Provides **antigenic specificity**
    - ■ **Two Classes**
      - ✓ Lipoteichoic acid: **spans PG** layer; **linked to plasma membrane**
      - ✓ Wall teichoic acid: **linked to PG** layer
- **Gram Negative (-) Cell Walls**
  - o <u>**Very few or one layer of PG and an outer membrane**</u>
  - o **PG** bonded to **lipoproteins** in the **outer membrane** and is in the **periplasm** (gel-like fluid between outer membrane and plasma membrane)
    - ■ **Outer membrane (OM):** phospholipids, lipoproteins, and **lipopolysaccharides (LPS)**
      - ✓ <u>**LPS component** important;</u> composed of
        - ❖ **Lipid A** (lipid portion): embedded in top layer of outer membrane; **an endotoxin**
        - ❖ **Core polysaccharide:** attached to Lipid A; contains unusual sugars; structural role
        - ❖ **O polysaccharide:** extends outward from core polysaccharide; composed of sugar molecules; **functions as an antigen**
      - ✓ **Porins** (proteins in membrane); **form channels;** permeability
  - o <u>**Do not have Techoic Acid**</u>; more susceptible to break

- **Cell Walls and the Gram Stain Mechanism/Stain/Color**
  - o **Crystal Violet (Primary stain):**
    - ■ **Gram (+):**   **Gram (-):**
  - o **Iodine (mordant):**
    - ■ **Gram (+):**   **Gram (-):**
  - o **Alcohol:**
    - ■ **Gram (+):**   **Gram (-):**
  - o **Safranin:**
    - ■ **Gram (+):**   **Gram (-):**

- **Atypical Cell Walls**
  - o **No walls or very little wall material**
    - ■ **Mycoplasma**
      - ✓ Smallest known bacteria
      - ✓ **Plasma membranes** made up of **sterols**
    - ■ **Archaea**

- ✓ **Lack** wall made of polysaccharides and proteins: **do not contain PG**
  - ■ **Acid Fast Cell Walls**
    - ✓ Mycolic Acid

F. Damage to Cell Wall
- ● **Bacterial cell wall** composition **different** from **eukaryotic cell walls**
- ● **Lysozyme** (an enzyme) located in **some eukaryotes (saliva, tears, mucus)**
  - o Active on most cell walls of **Gram (+)** bacteria
  - o Breaks the bonds of the disaccharides (NAG, NAM)→**lyses**
  - o **Contents** surrounded by the **plasma membrane** remaining intact **called:**
  - o **Protoplast: wall-less, spherical ; still carry out metabolic processes**
    - ■ **L forms:** lose their cell walls; **swell into irregularly shaped cells**
    - ■ **Spheroplast:** produced by **some Gram (-) cells;** consist: **of cellular contents, plasma membrane, some outer wall layer**
- ● **Protoplasts and Spherplasts**
  - o Burst in pure H_2O or dilute sugar or salt solutions: called **osmotic lyses**

G. Structures Internal to the Cell Wall
- ● **Plasma (Cytoplasmic) Membrane**
  - o **Encloses** the cytoplasm; provides a **barrier; selectively permeable**
  - o Lack **sterols;** less rigid than eukaryotes
  - o **Bilayer of phospholipids and proteins**
    - ■ **Nonpolar part: share electrons of atoms equally**
      - ✓ Two (2) tails (fatty acids); hydrophobic
    - ■ **Polar part: share electrons unequally**
      - ✓ Head (phosphate group and glycerol); hydrophilic
      - ✓ Face water surfaces (ECF and ICF)
    - ■ **Membrane Proteins**
      - ✓ **Integral Proteins**
        - ❖ Penetrate membrane completely
          - ***Transmembrane protein:** regulates movement of molecules thru membrane
          - ***Channel protein:** form pores or channels
      - ✓ **Peripheral Proteins**
        - *Lie at **inner and outer surface**
        - *May function as **enzymes, support**
  - o **Fluid Mosaic Model**
    - ■ Describes the structure of the plasma membrane
    - ■ Proteins are arranged in a **mosaic pattern**
    - ■ The membrane proteins and lipids flow freely within the plasma membrane
    - ■ **Regulate flow of molecules (nutrients) into cell and remove waste from cell**
  - o Main function: **Selectively permeable**
  - o Important in breakdown of nutrients and production of ATP
    - ■ **Chromatophores or thylakoids**
  - o **Mesosomes**
    - ■ Large, irregular folds; artifacts due to processing for EM
  - o Agents damaging plasma embrane
    - ■ Alcohols, QUAT's, polymyxins
- ● **Movement of Materials across Plasma (Cytoplasmic) Membranes**
  - o Substances cross the membrane by two processes
    - ■ **Passive Transport:** moves substances **into and out** of cell down a [] gradient **without ATP**

- ✓ **Simple Diffusion: net movement of substances from high [] to low []**; reach **equilibrium;** even distribution (oxygen, carbon dioxide)
- ✓ **Facilitated Diffusion: movement from high [] to low [] with assistance of an integral protein** (transporter) across a selectively permeable membrane (glucose)
- ✓ **Osmosis: diffusion of a solvent molecule from an area of high [] to an area of low []**
  - ❖ **Isotonic: same [] of solute and solvent;** equal movement of substances in and out cell
  - ❖ **Hypertonic: placed in environment** where there is **a high [] of solute;** water moves out of cell→**shrinkage;** plasmolysis
  - ❖ **Hypotonic: more solute [] inside cell,** water moves into cell→ **swelling;** osmotic lysis
  - ❖ Osmotic Pressure: **pressure** required to **prevent** movement of **pure water** into a solution containing some solutes
  - ■ **Active Transport: uses** energy **(ATP)** provided by cell, to move a substance across the membrane
    - ✓ Depends on **intergral membrane protein**
    - ✓ **Group Translocation:** a type of active transport that **modifies a substance; once substance passes through, membrane becomes impermeable** (glucose)
    - ✓ **Endocytosis:** form of **active transport;** eukaryotic cells; **large substances enter cell**
      - ❖ **Phagocytosis: engulfs solid** substances
      - ❖ **Pinocytosis: engulfs liquid** substances
    - ✓ **Exocytosis: process to remove large substances thru vesicles**
- ● **Cytoplasm**
  - o Substance of cell inside the plasma membrane; **aqueous, semitransparent**
  - o Waste, proteins, carbohydrates, lipids, inorganic ions, enzymes, water, small molecules
  - o Contains: for example (nucleoid, ribosomes, inclusions)
- ● **Nucleoid**
  - o **Bacterial chromosome: single, continuous, circular thread of ds DNA**
  - o **NOT** surrounded by a nuclear **envelope**
  - o **Chromosome attached** to plasma (cytoplasmic) membrane
  - o **No histones**
  - o Often contain **plasmids:** smaller, circular ds DNA; **extrachromosomal genetic elements;** not connected to main bacterial chromosome; replicate independently
- ● **Ribosomes**
  - o **Sites of protein synthesis**
  - o Comprised of **two subunits;** each consisting of **protein and ribosomal RNA (rRNA)**
  - o Prokaryotic ribosomes **differ** from eukaryotic ribosomes **in the # of proteins and rRNA molecules**
  - o Prokaryotes **smaller and less dense** than eukaryotes
  - o Identified by their sedimentation rate (mass, size, shape) **S=Svedberg/units**
  - o **Prokaryotes: 70S (Subunits: 30S and 50S); eukaryotes: 80S (Subunits: 40S and 60S)**
  - o Target for certain antibiotics: streptomycin, erythromycin
- ● **Inclusions**
  - o **Storage areas** for lipids, phosphate, starches, sulphur, nitrogen within the cytoplasm
    - ■ **Metachromatic Granules (aka Volutin)**
      - ✓ Stain red with a blue dye (methylene blue)
      - ✓ **Volutin:** reserve of **inorganic phosphate;** can be used in the synthesis of ATP
      - ✓ Formed by cells that grow in phosphate-rich environments
      - ✓ *Corynebacterium diptheriae* (diptheria)
    - ■ **Polysaccharide Granules**

- ✓ Consists **of glycogen and starch**
- ✓ When stained with **iodine granules** appear **blue**
  - ■ **Lipid Inclusions**
    - ✓ Stores **lipids**
    - ✓ Identified using **fat soluble dyes**
  - ■ **Sulfur Granules**
    - ✓ Serve as an **energy reserve**
  - ■ **Carboxysomes**
    - ✓ Contain the enzyme **ribulose 1,5-diphosphate carboxylase**
    - ✓ Used by **photosynthetic bacteria** for carbon dioxide fixation
  - ■ **Gas Vacuoles**
    - ✓ Contains **gas vesicles;** maintains **buoyancy**
  - ■ **Magetosomes**
    - ✓ Contains **iron oxide;** acts like a **magnet;** may **protect** against hydrogen peroxide accumulation

- ● **Endospores**
  - o Specialized **"resting or dormant"** cells
  - o Formed when **nutrients are removed** or depleted
  - o Certain **gram positive (+)** (*Clostridium, Bacillus*) and **gram negative (-)** (*Coxiella burnetii*) **bacteria**
  - o **Dehydrated** cells **with thick walls**
  - o **Formed internal** to bacterial cell membrane
  - o Survive extreme heat, lack of H_2O, toxic chemicals, radiation
  - o Process of **endospore** formation called **Sporulation or Sporogenesis**
    - ■ Begins in a **vegetative (parent) cell; nutrient(s)** unavailable
      - ✓ Newly replicated bacterial **DNA** and portion of **cytoplasm** isolated by ingrowth of plasma membrane; ingrowth called **spore septum**
      - ✓ **Spore septum** becomes double-layered; **surrounds chromosome** and **cytoplasm** forming a **forespore**
      - ✓ Layers of **peptidoglycan** laid down **between membrane**
      - ✓ Thick **spore coat** forms around **outside membrane; spore coat** responsible for resistance to harsh chemical surrounding
      - ✓ **Parent (vegetative)** cell degraded; **endospore freed**
  - o **Do not carry out metabolic reactions**
  - o Contains **dipicolinic acid (DPA)** protects **endospore DNA** from damage
  - o Dehydrated **endospore core** contains **only DNA, some RNA, ribosomes, enzymes,** important molecules; all important in **resuming metabolism** later
  - o Can remain **dormant** for years
  - o Can be located: **terminally** (at one end), **subterminally** (near one end), **centrally** (center)
  - o **Endospores** return to **vegetative state** by process called **Germination**
    - ■ Triggered by **damage to endospore's coat**
      - ✓ **Endospore enzymes** break down layers surrounding endospore
      - ✓ Water enters→**metabolism begins**
  - o **Sporulation or sporogenesis** in <u>**bacteria NOT a means of reproduction!!!!!!**</u>
  - o **Sporulation or sporogenesis** by **prokaryotic actinomycetes** and **eukaryotic fungi and algae** detach from parent and develop into another organism which is **reproduction**

H. The Eukaryotic Cells
- ● Consists of **animals, plants, algae, fungi, protozoa**
- ● **More complex structurally** than prokaryotes; **(highly organized)**
- ● Contain **"organelles"** which are **membrane bound;** perform **specialized function in cells metabolism**
- ● Contain **membrane bound nucleus**

- **Flagella and Cilia**
  - **Flagella** (singular: **flagellum**)
    - Some **have flagella;** usually **few** and **long;** moves in **wavelike manner**
  - **Cilia** (singular: **cilium**)
    - Projections **numerous** and **short**; move material along surface of cells
  - **Flagella and Cilia**
    - Both used for **locomotion**
    - Both **anchored to plasma membrane** by a **basal body**
    - Both consist of **9 pairs of microtubules** (in a ring) plus **two microtubules** (in center) **called 9 + 2 array**
    - **Microtubules** made up of protein **tubulin**
- **Cell Wall and Glycocalyx**
  - **Cell Wall**
    - **Most** eukaryotes **have cell walls; simpler** than prokaryotes
    - Composition differs with each organism
      - ✓ **Chitin**: principle component of most fungi
      - ✓ **Cellulose**: many algae, plants, some fungi
      - ✓ **Glucan and mannan**: yeasts
      - ✓ Outer **Protein (pellicle), no cell wall**: protozoa
    - Eukaryotic cells **do not contain peptidoglycans**
  - **Glycocalyx**
    - Covers plasma membrane; made of **sticky carbohydrates**
    - Can form **lipoproteins and glycolipids**
    - Gives cell **strength**; help cell **to adhere to other cells**
- **Plasma (Cytoplasm) Membrane**
  - Very similar in function and structure to prokaryotic cells
  - **Selectively permeable;** encloses cytoplasm of the cell
  - Barrier between the inner cell and its environment
  - Contain **sterols** (complex lipids); helps **prevent destruction** of cell membrane **from increased osmotic pressure**
  - Can act as **Pseudopods** (false feet) in certain eukaryotes ; extensions of the plasma membrane; **movement**
  - Perform mechanism of **Endocytosis: surround, enclose, bring into cell** a particle or large molecule
  - **Three** types of **Endocytosis**
    - **Pinocytosis**: bring in **extracellular fluid**
    - **Phagocytosis**: pseudopods engulf **particles;** used by white blood cells
    - **Receptor-mediated endocytosis**: substances **bind to receptors** in membrane; membrane folds in
- **Cytoplasm**
  - Contains cytosol (fluid portion), organelles, inclusions, **Cytoskeleton**
  - **Cytoskeleton**: consist of **microfilaments, intermediate filaments, microtubules;** provides **support** and **shape**
  - Movement of cytoplasm from one part of cell to another part **called cytoplasmic streaming;** helps distribute nutrients and move the cell

H. The Eukaryotic Cells
- **Ribosomes**
  - **Site of protein synthesis**
  - Can be **free (unattached):** synthesize proteins used for inside cell

21

- o Can be **attached** (to nuclear membrane or endoplasmic reticulum)**:** synthesize proteins destined for insertion in plasma membrane or export
- o **Larger and denser** than prokaryotic cells
- o **80S consist of large 60S** (three molecules of rRNA) and **smaller 40S** (one molecule of rRNA)
- o Chloroplasts and mitochondria contain 70S ribosomes
- o Mitochondrial ribosomes synthesize mitochondrial proteins
- o **Polysomes:** 10 to 20 ribosomes join together
- **Nucleus** (pleural: **nuclei**)
  - o Oval or round in shape
  - o **Contains DNA** which is contained **within a nuclear envelope**
  - o **Nuclear pores allows the nucleus to communicate with the cytoplasm**
  - o **DNA** is combined with several proteins including **histones** and nonhistones
  - o **DNA** (165 bps) and **histones** (9 molecules) make **a nucleosome**
  - o Cell at rest **(not reproducing)** forms **chromatin: DNA + proteins appear as a threadlike mass**
  - o Dividing cell **(nuclear division) forms chromosomes: threads of chromatin condense and coil (rod shaped)**
- **Nucleolus** (plural: **nucleoli**)
  - o Within nuclear envelope
  - o Condensed regions of chromosomes where ribosomal RNA **(rRNA) synthesis** occurs
- **Endoplasmic Reticulum (ER)**
  - o Continuous with the **nuclear envelope**
  - o Contributes to the support and distribution of the cytoplasm
  - o **Pathway for transporting lipids and proteins**
  - o Stores lipid and proteins until needed by cell
  - o Consist of **cisterns (network of flattened membranous sacs) filled** with **proteins or lipids** that are **"packaged";** detach from the Golgi Complex; transported to another part of the cell
  - o **Two distinct forms of ER**
    - ■ rough ER (RER):covered by ribosomes (sites for protein synthesis); continuous with nuclear envelope; factory for **synthesizing secretory proteins and membrane molecules**
    - ■ smooth ER (SER):extends from RER; **not covered by ribosomes; site for phospholipid, fats, and steroids synthesis**
- **Golgi Complex**
  - o Considered the **"FEDEX SYSTEM"** of the cell
  - o **Packages and delivers proteins throughout the cell and the environment**
  - o Contains **cisterns** (curved shaped) **stacked on top of each other**
  - o Portion of **ER membrane buds off with proteins (synthesized by ribosomes)** forming a **transport vesicle**
  - o **Vesicle fuses** with a **cistern of the Golgi Complex**
  - o Release **proteins into the cistern**
  - o **Proteins "modified"**
  - o Move from one cistern to another via **transfer vesicles** that bud from the edge of the cistern
  - o Enzymes inside cisternae **modify the proteins** to form glycoproteins, glycolipids, lipoproteins
  - o Some of the **"processed"** proteins leave the cisterns in **secretory vesicles**
  - o **Secretory vesicles** detach from the cistern; deliver the **"modified"** proteins to the plasma membrane where they are **discharged by exocytosis**
  - o **Some "processed"** proteins leave cistern in **storage vesicles (lysosomes)**
- **Lysosomes**
  - o Have **a single membrane; lack internal structures**
  - o Contain **digestive enzymes** able to digest molecules, bacteria
- **Mitochondria** (singular: **mitochondrion**)

- o Oval or rod shaped
- o Power house of the cell (**ATP production**)
- o **Double membrane structure**
    - ■ **Outer: smooth**
    - ■ **Inner: arranged in folds** called **cristae** (singular:**crista**)
        - ✓ **Cristae: contain** enzyme making ATP and some proteins functioning in cellular respiration located here
- o **Center** filled with semi fluid substance called **matrix**
- o Contain: **70S ribosomes;** some **DNA** of their own; machinery necessary for replication, transcription, and translation of their own **DNA**
- o Can **reproduce** more or less on its own by growing and dividing in two
- ● **Chloroplasts**
    - o Located in **green plants and algae**
    - o **Membrane-enclosed structure;** contains **chlorophyll** and **enzymes** needed **for "photosynthesis"**
    - o **Chlorophyll** contained **in sacs** (called **thylakoids**)
    - o Stacks **of thylakoids** called **grana** (singular: **granum**)
    - o Like mitochondria **contains:** 70S ribosomes, DNA, enzymes involved in protein synthesis
    - o Multiply on their own within the cell **by increasing in size, then divide in two**
- ● **Peroxisomes**
    - o Similar in structure to lysosomes but smaller
    - o Contain **1 or more enzymes** which can **"oxidize"** certain organic substances
    - o Contain **catalase**
- ● **Vacuoles**
    - o Derived **from Golgi Complex**
    - o **Space** in cytoplasm **enclosed by** membrane called **a tonoplast**
    - o **Storage for:** proteins, sugar, organic acid; takes up H_2O; brings in food
- ● **Centriole**
    - o **Pair of cylindrical structures** near the nucleus
    - o Composed of **nine clusters of three microtubules (triplets)** arranged **in a circular pattern called 9+0 array** (*9* cluster of microtubules and *0* microtubules in the center)
    - o Plays a part in **eukaryotic cell division**
- ● **Centrosome**
    - o Located near the nucleus; consists **of two components**
        - ■ **Pericentriolar area (or material):** region of cytosol; **composed** of dense network of small **protein fibers; organizing center for mitotic spindle; important in cell division**
        - ■ **Centrioles: within the pericentriolar space;** a pair of cylindrical structures

I. Endosymbiotic Theory

- ● **Explains the origin of eukaryotes from prokaryotes**
    - o Larger bacterial cells engulfed smaller bacterial cells; one living within another called **endosymbiosis**
    - o **Ancestral eukaryote developed a rudimentary nucleus when plasma membrane surrounded the chromosome**
    - o The cell now called a **nucleoplasm,** may have engulfed **an aerobic bacteria**
    - o This bacteria lived in a symbiotic relationship where host nucleoplasm supplied nutrients for bacterium
    - o Endosymbiotic bacterium produced energy that could be used by the nucleoplasm
    - o **Chloroplasts may be descendents of photosynthetic prokaryotes** ingested by the **nucleoplasm**

MICROBIOLOGY

MICROBIAL METABOLISM

A. Catabolic and Anabolic Reactions
- **Metabolism**
  - **The sum of all chemical reactions within a living organism**
  - Divided into 2 classes
    - **Catabolism: breakdown or degrading** of complex organic compounds into simpler ones
      - ✓ Generally hydrolytic
      - ✓ **Exergonic:** produce more energy than consumed
    - **Anabolism: build** complex organic molecules from simpler ones
      - ✓ Involve dehydration synthesis reactions
      - ✓ **Endergonic:** consume more energy than produced
  - *Catabolic reactions provide building blocks for anabolic reactions made possible through **ATP***
  - **ATP stores energy** received from catabolic reactions **and releases energy** later to drive anabolic reactions

    ATP→ ADP + P + energy

    ADP + P +energy → ATP

B. Enzymes
- **Proteins** involved in chemical reactions
- Determines a cells metabolic pathway
- **Collision Theory**
  - Explains how chemical reactions occur and how certain factors affect the rate of these reactions
  - **Everything (atoms, molecules) continually moving and colliding with each other**. This can cause chemical bonds to be formed or broken
  - Factors which determine a "collision" to cause a reaction include
    - **Velocity**
    - **Energy of the colliding particles**
    - **Configuration**
  - **Activation energy: the amount** of energy needed to **"break up"** the stable electronic configuration, so electrons can be rearranged
  - **Reaction rate is the "frequency"** of collisions containing enough energy to bring about a reaction
    - Reaction rate depends on the number of reactant molecules at or greater than the activation energy level
    - Reaction rate can be **increased by**
      - ✓ Increase **in temperature** will raise the rate
      - ✓ Increase **in pressure** will cause an increase in collisions
      - ✓ Increase **in concentration**, of reactants, will cause an increase in collisions
- In living cells, **enzymes** act as <u>**biological catalyst**</u>: substances which speed up a chemical reaction **without** being permanently changed or altered
- As a **catalyst,** each **enzyme** acts on a specific substance called **"substrate"** catalyzing one reaction
  - Example: sucrose _____→ **glucose + fructose**

Sucrase

- **Enzymes** have a **3-D shape** with **region** which **interacts** with the **substrate** called **"active site"**
- **The enzyme-substrate-complex (ESC)**
  o Formed by the **temporary binding of enzyme and reactants**
  o Allows the **collisions to be more effective** and **lowers the activation energy** of the reaction
- **Have specificity and efficiency**
  o Possible by their shape (**configuration**)
  o **Enzymes** are large globular proteins with **a 3-D shape**
  o **Configuration** helps to "find" the **correct substrate** among large numbers of different molecules
  o **Enzymes** extremely **efficient**; catalyze reactions at very high rates
- **Naming enzymes**
  o Usually end in **-ase**
  o **Grouped in classes** according to the **type of chemical reaction they catalyze**
- **Enzyme components**
  o **Some** enzymes consist **entirely of proteins**
  o **Most** enzymes consist of
    ■ **A protein portion (Apoenzyme): inactive; activated by cofactors**
    ■ **A non-protein portion (Cofactor)**
      ✓ If cofactor is an *organic molecule* called **coenzyme**
      ✓ Some **coenzymes** act as **electron carriers**
      ✓ Many **coenzymes** are derived from **vitamins**
  o **Holoenzyme: apoenzyme + cofactor**
- **Mechanism of enzymatic action**
  o Enzymes lower the activation energy of chemical reactions
  o **Sequence of events**
    ■ **Active site:** substrate contacts specific region of the enzyme
    ■ **ESC:** temporary intermediate compound forms
    ■ **Transformation:** substrate is transformed by rearranging of existing atoms
    ■ **Transformed substrate molecule (product):** released
    ■ **Unchanged enzyme:** free to react again
- **Factors influencing enzymatic activity**
  o **Temperature**
    ■ Increases rate at an optimum temperature
    ■ **Beyond** optimum temperature **leads to denaturation** (breaks hydrogen and noncovalent bonds)
  o **pH**
    ■ **Most** enzymes have **an optimum pH**
    ■ **Extreme** changes can **cause denaturation**
  o **Substrate concentration**
    ■ When the [] of substrate (s) is extremely high can a maximum rate be attained
    ■ **High substrate concentration** (when all active sites occupied) the **enzyme is saturated**
  o **Inhibitors**
    ■ Control **enzymes**
      ✓ **Competitive Inhibitors**
        ❖ **Fill active site; "compete"** with normal substrate
          *Bind **irreversibly:** won't let go!
          *Bind **reversibly:** bind and leave; slows interaction with substrate
      ✓ **Noncompetitive Inhibitors**
        ❖ **Interact** with **another part** of the enzyme (**allosteric site**)
        ❖ Cause **"active site"** to **change shape** (nonconform)
        ❖ Irreversible or Reversible

- Feedback (or end-product) Inhibition
  - A series of enzymes make an end product
  - End product inhibits first enzyme in the series
  - Process shuts down the entire pathway when enough end product is made
- Ribozymes
  - Unique type of RNA: functions as a *catalyst,* have active sites that bind substrates
  - Specifically act on strands of RNA by removing sections and splicing the remaining pieces

C. Energy (ATP) Production
- <u>Two</u> general aspects of energy production
  - Oxidation-Reduction Reactions
    - Oxidation-removal of electrons (e-) from an atom or molecule; produces energy
    - Reduction-gain 1 or > electrons
    - *Oxidation-reduction reactions <u>always</u> coupled; <u>redox reaction</u>*
  - Generation of ATP
    - Most energy released during redox reactions are trapped in the cell by the formation of ATP
    - ADP + Energy + P→ATP
    - Addition of P called phosphorylation
    - Three mechanisms of phosphorylation to generate ATP from ADP
      - ✓ Substrate-Level Phosphorylation
        - ❖ ATP generated when high energy phosphate group (P) is directly transferred from a phosphorylated compound to ADP
      - ✓ Oxidative Phosphorylation
        - ❖ Electrons transferred from organic compounds to one group of electron carriers (NAD+, FAD)
        - ❖ The electrons are passed through a series of different carriers to molecules of oxygen or other inorganic and organic molecules
        - ❖ Sequence of electron carriers uses called the electron transport chain (ETC)
      - ✓ Photophosphorylation
        - ❖ In photosynthetic cells which contain the light-trapping pigments like chlorophylls
        - ❖ Converts light energy to chemical energy of ATP and NADPH
        - ❖ ATP and NADPH used to synthesize organic molecules
        - ❖ ETC involved, also

D. Metabolic Pathways of Energy Production
- A series of enzymatically catalyzed chemical reactions which store and release energy from organic molecules
- Carbohydrate Catabolism
  - Breakdown of carbohydrate molecules to produce energy
  - The main energy source of metabolic reactions
  - Glucose most common carbohydrate source used by cells
  - To produce energy from glucose, two processes used
    - Cellular respiration
    - Fermentation
    - Both usually start with first step: <u>*Glycolysis*</u>
  - *Glycolysis (Embden-Meyerhof Pathway)*
    - Pathway of ten chemical reactions; each catalyzed by a different enzyme
    - Can occur if oxygen is present or not

- Consist of **two basic stages**
  - ✓ **Preparatory stage:** two molecules of ATP are used to split a 6-carbon glucose molecule into two three-carbon compounds (GP) and (DHAP)
  - ✓ **Energy-conserving stage:** the three-carbon molecules are oxidized to 2-molecules of **pyruvic acid**; four molecules of ATP formed
  - **Glucose** broken down into **two molecules of pyruvic acid**
- **Carbohydrate Catabolism (Cont.)**
  - o **Alternatives to glycolysis**
    - **The Pentose phosphate Pathway:** metabolize 5-carbon sugars
    - **Entner-Doudoroff Pathway:** metabolize glucose without glycolysis or pentose phosphate pathway; certain bacteria lack certain enzymes essential for glycolysis (ex:phosphofructokinase-1)

E. Cellular Respiration
  - After glucose broken down to **pyruvic acid**, the **pyruvic acid** funneled into the next step of either **cellular respiration** or **fermentation**
    - o **Cellular Respiration:** ATP generating process; molecules oxidized; **final electron acceptor** is almost always **an inorganic molecule**; essential feature is **operation of an ETC**
    - o **Two types of Cellular Respiration**
      - **Aerobic:** uses **oxygen**; final electron acceptor is **oxygen**
      - **Anaerobic:** does not use oxygen; final electron acceptor is **an inorganic molecule** or rarely **an organic molecule**
    - o **Aerobic Respiration (Krebs cycle, TCA cycle, citric acid cycle)**
      - Uses **oxygen**; final electron acceptor is **oxygen**
      - Series of **biochemical reactions** in which potential chemical **energy stored in acetyl CoA is released**
      - Series of oxidation and reduction reactions **transfer the potential energy** (in the form of electrons) **to electron carrier coenzymes**
      - **Pyruvic acid is decarboxylated** (to enter the Kreb Cycle) producing one CO_2 molecule and **one acetyl group**
      - **Two-carbon acetyl groups oxidized;** electrons picked up by **NAD+ and FAD for ETC**
      - From one molecule of glucose, oxidation produces: six molecules of NADPH, two molecules of FADH2, two molecules of ATP
      - Decarboxylation produces **six molecules of CO_2**
      - Electrons brought to the ETC by **NADH**
      - **ETC** consists of carriers
      - **Protons** pumped across the membrane generate a **"force"** as electrons move through a series of acceptors or carriers
      - **Chemiosmotic Mechanism of ATP generation:** explains the mechanism of ATP synthesis using the ETC; concentration gradients (**diffusion**) yields energy, **active transport** yields energy
      - The energy produced from this **movement used by *ATP synthase* to make ATP from ADP and P**
      - **In eukaryotic cells:** electron carriers located **in the inner mitochondria membrane**
        - ✓ **36 ATP molecules produced**
      - **In prokaryotic cells:** carriers located **in the plasma membrane**
        - ✓ **38 ATP molecules produced**
    - o **Anaerobic Respiration**
      - Does not use oxygen; **final electron acceptor is an inorganic substance**
      - **Total ATP** yield is less **because parts of the Krebs cycle operates under anaerobic conditions**

F. Fermentation

- **Pyruvic acid converted to an organic product;** NAD+ and NADP+ regenerated
- **Does not require oxygen; does not use an ETC system or Krebs cycle; occurs in cytoplasm!!**
- Uses an organic molecule as the final electron acceptor; produces small amounts of ATP
- **Lactic acid fermentation: the pyruvic acid is reduced to lactic acid by NADH**
- **Alcohol fermentation: acetaldehyde is reduced to ethanol by NADH**

G. Metabolic Pathways of Energy Production

- **Lipid Catabolism**
  - **Lipases** hydrolyze lipids into glycerol and fatty acids (FA's)
  - In glycolysis the FA's are broken down by beta-oxidation
  - The catabolic products can be further broken down in glycolysis and Krebs cycle
- **Protein Catabolism**
  - Proteins too large to cross plasma membrane
  - Microorganism secretes **protease and peptidases** to split proteins into amino acids (aa's)
  - The aa's undergo deamination, decarboxylation, dehydrogenation reactions to enter Krebs Cycle

H. Biochemical Tests

- Used to identify microbes (bacteria, yeast) in the laboratory; **detect the presence or absence of enzymes**
  - Detects certain amino acid catabolizing enzymes
  - Catabolize certain carbohydrates
  - Catabolize and produce acid
  - Produce gas
  - Identify bacteria which cause disease; presence or absence of ETC
- **Different microbes produce different enzymes**

I. Photosynthesis

- **The ability for some organisms to synthesize complex organic compounds from inorganic substances**
- Carried out by many microbes and plants
- The chemical conversion of light energy (from the sun) into chemical energy
$$6CO_2 + 12 H_2O + light \rightarrow C_6H_{12}O_6 + 6O_2 + 6H_2O$$
- The energy from the sunlight is used to reduce CO_2 to carbohydrates
- Need **chlorophyll** (light-sensitive pigment)
- Summarized as follows:
  - **Plants, algae, cyanobacteria:** use water as a hydrogen donor, releasing oxygen
$$6CO_2 + 12 H_2O + light\ energy \rightarrow C_6H_{12}O_6 + 6H_2O + 6O2$$
  - **Purple sulfur and green sulfur bacteria:** use H_2S as a hydrogen donor, producing sulfur granules
$$6CO_2 + 12 H_2O + light\ energy \rightarrow C_6H_{12}O_6 + 6H_2O + 12 S$$
- Takes place in two stages
  - **Light-dependent (light) reactions**
    - Light energy used to convert ADP and P to ATP
    - $NADP^+$ reduced to NADPH
    - NADPH is an energy-rich carrier of electrons
    - Mechanism used is *Photophosphorylation*
      - ✓ Light energy absorbed by chlorophyll in the cell→excitation of some molecules' electrons

28

    ✓ Electrons from chlorophyll pass through an ETC system where ATP is produced by **chemiosmosis**

    ✓ Contain **photosystems**
- ❖ Consist of chlorophyll and other pigments packed in thylakoid membranes
- ❖ Sensitive to certain wavelengths

    ✓ **Cyclic photophosphorylation:** electrons return to the chlorophyll; energy converted to ATP

    ✓ **Noncyclic photophosphorylation:** electrons do not return to chlorophyll; become incorporated into NADPH; products are ATP, O_2, and NADPH

- o **Light-independent (dark) reactions**
  - ■ Require no light directly
  - ■ NADPH used along with energy from ATP to reduce CO_2 to sugar
  - ■ Includes **Calvin-Benson Cycle:** CO_2 used to synthesize sugars

J. Summary of Energy Production Mechanisms

- ● Energy passes from one organism to another in the form of potential energy in the bonds of chemical compounds
- ● The energy obtained for organisms from oxidation-reduction reactions
- ● Need electron donor(s) as initial energy source in cell
- ● Electrons removed from the chemical energy sources transferred to electron carriers (some ATP produced)
- ● Electrons then transferred from carrier to final electron acceptor, producing more ATP
  - o Aerobic respiration: O_2 final electron acceptor
  - o Anaerobic respiration: inorganic substances serve as final electron acceptor
  - o Aerobic and anaerobic respiration: ETC used to synthesize ATP
  - o Fermentation: organic compounds serve as final electron acceptor

K. Energy and Carbon Sources for Microbes

- ● Classified metabolically according to their nutritional pattern (**sources of energy and carbon**)
  - o **Energy sources**
    - ■ **Phototrophs:** use **light** as primary energy source
    - ■ **Chemotrophs:** depend on **oxidation-reductions** reactions **of inorganic or organic compounds**
  - o **Carbon sources**
    - ■ **Autotrophs** (self-feeders) or *lithotrophs*: use CO_2
    - ■ **Heterotrophs** (feeders on others) or *organotrophs*: require an organic carbon source
      - ✓ Further classified according to their source of **organic molecules**
        - ❖ **Saprophytes:** dead organic material
        - ❖ Parasites: from living host
- ● If we **combine energy and carbon sources**, we can identify organisms by **nutritional classifications**
  - o **Photoautotrophs**
    - ■ Use **light** (energy) and CO_2 (carbon source)
    - ■ Green plants, algae, green and purple bacteria, cyanobacteria
    - ■ Oxygenic: photosynthetic process **produces O_2**
    - ■ Anoxygenic: process **does not produce O_2**
  - o **Photoheterotrophs**
    - ■ Use **light** (energy) and **organic compounds: alcohols, FA's, other carbs (carbon source)**
    - ■ Green and purple nonsulfur bacteria
    - ■ Anoxygenic

- o **Chemoautotrophs**
  - Use **electrons from reduced inorganic compounds (energy)** and **CO_2 (carbon source)**
  - Hydrogen, sulfur, iron, nitrogen, and carbon monoxide oxidizing bacteria
- o **Chemoheterotrophs**
  - *Energy and carbon source are usually same complex organic molecule* (ex. Glucose)
  - Use the electrons from hydrogen atoms in organic compounds as their energy source
  - Animals, fungi, protozoa, bacteria

L. Metabolic Pathways of Energy Use
- *Synthesis* of molecules **requires energy**
- Microbes can use ATP for motion (flagella), active transport (across plasma membrane), making cellular components
  - o **Polysaccharide Biosynthesis**
    - Microbes synthesize sugars and polysaccharides
    - Glycogen, peptidoglycan
  - o **Lipid Biosynthesis**
    - Lipids synthesized from fatty acids and glycerol
    - Structural components of biological membranes, provide pigments, energy storage
  - o **Amino Acid and Protein Biosynthesis**
    - Most amino acids needed for protein synthesis
    - Amino acids can be synthesized directly or indirectly from intermediates of carbohydrate metabolism (Krebs cycle)
    - Proteins play role in cell as enzymes, structural components, toxins
  - o **Purine and Pyrimidine Biosynthesis**
    - DNA and RNA consist of repeating nucleotides which consist of purine or pyrimidine, pentose, phosphate group
    - Carbon and nitrogen atoms from certain amino acids form the backbone of purines and pyrimidines

M. Integration of Metabolism
- Anabolic and Catabolic reactions are integrated through a group of common intermediates
- Anabolic and Catabolic reactions share some metabolic pathways
- Metabolic pathways functioning in anabolism and catabolism called **amphibolic pathways**

MICROBIOLOGY

MICROBIAL GROWTH

A. Requirements for Growth
- Refers to **number of cells, not size**
- Divided into **two main categories**
  - **Physical Requirements**
    - Includes **temperature, pH, osmotic pressure**
    - **Temperature**
      - ✓ Most organisms grow well in temperatures favored by humans
      - ✓ Five groups based on preferred temperature range
        - ❖ **Psychrophiles: cold-loving** (-10° to 20°) C; optimum 15° C; ocean's depth; polar regions
        - ❖ **Psychrotrophs:** (0° to 30°) C; optimum 10° to 20° C; grow well at refrigerator temperatures
        - ❖ **Mesophiles: moderate temperatures** (10° to 50°); (optimum 25° C to 40°C); **most common type of microbe**
        - ❖ **Thermophiles: heat (40° to 70°) C**; optimum 50°C to 60°C; organic compost
        - ❖ **Hyperthermophiles: extreme heat**; optimum 80° C or >; hot springs
      - ✓ Each bacterial species grow best within a limited range
      - ✓ Each species grows poorly at extreme high and low temperatures within their range
        - ❖ **Minimum growth Temperature:** lowest temperature it will grow
        - ❖ **Optimum growth Temperature:** grows best
        - ❖ **Maximum growth Temperature:** highest temperature which growth is possible
      - ✓ **Refrigeration** is the **most common method to preserve foods;** slows growth rate
    - **pH**
      - ✓ Refers to acidity or alkalinity of a solution
      - ✓ **Most bacteria grow best near neutrality (pH 6.5 to 7.5)**
      - ✓ Few grow in acidic pH (below **4.0**)
        - ❖ **Acidophiles:** tolerant to acidity
        - ❖ **Molds and yeast:** optimum **pH 5 to 6**
    - **Osmotic Pressure**
      - ✓ Refers to the minimum pressure applied to a solution to prevent inward flow of water across a semipermeable membrane
      - ✓ Microorganisms get most of their nutrients from surrounding water
      - ✓ **High osmotic pressure removes water from cell**
        - ❖ **Hypertonic solution:** solution whoses concentration of **solutes (solid, liquid, gas)** is higher outside the cell; allows cellular water to leave through plasma membrane to the high solute concentration; called **plasmolysis (or shrinkage of cytoplasm)**
        Ex: high sugar or salt concentrations
          - *Extreme halophiles (obligate halophiles): adapt to high salt solutions (30% salt)
          - *Facultative halophiles: grow at salt concentrations up to 2% to 15%
        - ❖ **Hypotonic solution:** solution which the concentration of **solutes** is lower outside the cell; allows cellular water to enter through the plasma membrane; called **turgid (lysed or swelling of cytoplasm)**

Ex: distilled water

- o **Chemical Requirements**
  - ■ **Water**
  - ■ **Carbon**
    - ✓ Structural backbone of living matter
    - ✓ Needed for **all organic compounds**
  - ■ **Nitrogen (N), Sulfur (S), Phosphorus (P)**
    - ✓ For protein synthesis **(N, S)**
    - ✓ For DNA and RNA synthesis **(N, P)**
    - ✓ For ATP synthesis **(P)**
    - ✓ **Nitrogen**
      - ❖ Primarily to form the amino group of the amino acids of proteins
      - ❖ Used in nitrogen fixation (use nitrogen gas directly from the atmosphere)
    - ✓ **Sulfur**
      - ❖ Used to synthesize sulfur-containing amino acids and vitamins (thiamine, biotin)
    - ✓ **Phosphorus**
      - ❖ Essential for synthesis of nucleic acids; phospholipids of cell membrane
      - ❖ Found in energy bonds of ATP
  - ■ **Trace Elements**
    - ✓ **Iron, copper, zinc, molybdenum**
    - ✓ Essential for the function of certain enzymes
  - ■ **Oxygen**
    - ✓ Microbes that use oxygen (aerobes) produce more energy from nutrients than microbes that do not use oxygen (anaerobes)
      - ❖ *Obligate aerobes*: **require oxygen to live**
      - ❖ *Facultative anaerobes*: **use oxygen when present; BUT can continue growth if oxygen not available** (by fermentation or anaerobic respiration); efficiency in producing energy decreases (E. Coli, many yeast)
      - ❖ *Obligate anaerobes*: **unable to use O_2; can be harmed by the presense of oxygen**
        (Clostridium-tetanus, botulism)
        *Toxic forms of oxygen causing harm to microbes:
        - ➢ **Singlet Oxygen**
          -Normal molecular oxygen
          -Pushed into **a higher-energy state** and is very reactive
        - ➢ **Superoxide Radicals (or superoxide anions)**
          -Small amounts formed during normal respiration of organisms that use O_2
          -**Obligate anaerobes,** in the presence of oxygen, **form superoxide radical** which is toxic; lack enzyme super oxide dismutase (SOD)
          -SOD, an enzyme, neutralize the radicals
          -Aerobic bacteria, facultative anaerobes growing aerobically, aero tolerant: all produce SOD
          -SOD converts the superoxide **radical into oxygen and hydrogen peroxide**
        - ➢ **Hydrogen Peroxide**
          -Contains a toxic peroxide anion
          -Hydrogen peroxide neutral**ized by catalase and peroxidase**
        - ➢ **The Hydroxyl Radical**
          -Very reactive
          -Formed in cellular cytoplasm

❧   *Obligate anaerobes:* **usually do not produce SOD or CATALASE**

❧   *Aerotolerant anaerobes:* **cannot use oxygen <u>for growth</u>,** but tolerate it well

     *Many ferment carbohydrates to lactic acid (lactobacilli)

     *Possess **SOD only**

❧   *Microaerophiles:* **aerobic; grow in low []'s of oxygen**

- **Organic Growth Factors**
  - ❧ Essential organic compounds in which the organism is **unable to synthesize; obtained from the environment**
  - ❧ Some bacteria lack the enzymes needed for the synthesis of certain vitamins

B. Biofilms

- Type of community in which microbes live in
- Reside in a **matrix** primarily of **polysaccharides**, DNA, and proteins called *slime*
- Also considered a **hydrogel**
- Have cell-to-cell chemical communication (or **quorum sensing**); share nutrients and protect
- Usually **attached to a surface**
- Can be a single species or diverse group of microbes
- Begins as a free-swimming (**planktonic**) bacterium attaching to a surface
- Important in human health; very resistant to microbicides
- Treated with antimicrobials agents which penetrate surface, or with lactoferrin

C. Culture Media

- **Nutrient material** prepared for **the growth of microorganisms** in a laboratory
- **Microorganisms introduced** into a culture medium to **initiate growth** called **inoculum**
- **Microbes that grow and multiply** refered to as **a culture**
- Initially sterile (**contain no living organisms**); will contain the inoculum and its offsprings
- Variety depends on species to be grown
- **Agar** (from a marine alga; a complex polysaccharide) added to produce a **solid medium**
  - o Can be placed in test tubes (**slants, deep**)
  - o Can be placed in shallow dishes (called **petri or culture plates** when filled)
- **Chemically Defined Media**
  - o Certain microbes unable to synthesize specific energy sources, carbon, nitrogen, sulfur, phosphorus, and any organic factors needed to grow; need a specific medium
  - o **Exact** chemical composition is known; **specific**
- **Complex Media**
  - o Made up of **nutrients including extracts from yeast, meat or plants, or digested proteins**
  - o **Varies** slightly from batch to batch
  - o The energy, carbon, nitrogen, sulfur requirements provided primarily by protein
  - o Vitamins and other organic growth factors provided from meat extracts
  - o **Nutrient broth**: liquid form
  - o **Nutrient agar**: agar added
    - ■ Agar is not a nutrient
- **Reducing Media**
  - o **Anaerobic growth media** used to grow anaerobic bacteria
  - o Contains ingredients like **sodium thioglycolate (combines and depletes O_2 in the medium)**
  - o Stored in tightly capped test tubes
  - o Heated before use (drives off O_2)
  - o To grow **anaerobes in Petri plates**, several methods available
    - ■ Incubate microbes in sealed boxes and jars; oxygen removed after culture plates introduced and the container is sealed

- Add water to certain chemicals which need a **catalyst;** produce hydrogen and carbon dioxide and remove the oxygen
- One system, no water or catalyst needed; active ingredient in its chemicals is **ascorbic acid**
- **Individual Petri plates** (Oxyplate) become an **anaerobic chamber;** *oxyrase*
- Anaerobic chambers for large volume of work; filled with inert gases and air locks
- **Special Culture Techniques**
    - Many bacteria, viruses **do not grow on artificial laboratory medium**
        - Armadillos (*Mycobacterium leprae*); living host cells (rickettsias, chlamydias)
    - Carbon dioxide incubators: **grow aerobic bacteria needing increased or decreased []'s to grow**
        - Candle jars: cultures placed in jar with lighted candle and sealed
        - Small plastic bags with self-contained chemical gas generators
        - **Capnophiles:** grow well at high CO_2 []'s (GI tract, respiratory tract)
    - Biosafely levels 1 ot 4 *(BSL 1to 4)*
        - Dangerous organisms
        - Precautions taken such as: special gloves, clothing, hoods, filtration, pressurization
- **Selective and Differential Media**
    - Helps detect the **presence of specific microbes** associated with disease or poor sanitation
        - **Selective Media**
            - ✓ **Suppress** the growth of **unwanted bacteria** and **encourage growth** of **wanted microbes**
            - ✓ Bismuth sulfite agar: Inhibits growth of gram (+) and most gram (-) intestinal bacteria (*Salmonella typhi* from feces)
            - ✓ Sabouraud's dextrose agar (pH 5.6): grows fungi
        - **Differential Media**
            - ✓ **Distinguishes colonies of desired organism from other colonies growing on same plate**
            - ✓ Blood agar (contains RBC's) identifies microbes that destroy RBC's
                - ❖ *Streptococcus pyogenes*: causes strep throat; produce **"clear ring"** around the colonies; called **beta-hemolysis)**
        - **Selective and Differential Combined**
            - ✓ Mannitol salt agar: contains high salt content and mannitol
                - ❖ Selected for *Staphylococcus aureus*
            - ✓ MacConkey agar: contains bile salts, crystal violet, lactose (inhibits gram positive (+)); certain gram negative (-) can be differentiated (Salmonella)
        - **Enrichment Culture**
            - ✓ Designed to **increase numbers of desired microbes** to detectable levels
            - ✓ Usually a liquid which provides nutrients and environmental conditions favorable for the growth of a particular microbe, but not others (soil, feces)
            - ✓ Chocolate agar

D. Obtaining Pure Cultures (or Clones)

- Forming the **exact copies** of the original organism
- **Colony** comes from **a single spore, cell, or group of the same microorganisms attached to one another**
- Method **most commonly used**
    - **Streak Plate Method**
        - Sterile inoculating loop dipped in mixed culture (containing more than one type of microorganism) and is *streaked* in a certain pattern over the medium; spreads colonies to grow individually

E. Preserving Bacterial Cultures
- **Methods for storage of cultures**
  - **Short term:** uses **refrigeration**
  - **Long term**
    - **Deep-freezing**
      - ✓ Pure culture place in a liquid and quick frozen (-50° C to -95° C)
      - ✓ Usually thawed and cultured
      - ✓ Last several years
    - **Lyophilization (freeze-drying)**
      - ✓ Quickly frozen (-54°C to -72°C) and H_2O removed by a high vacumn
      - ✓ Under vacumn, container sealed by melting the glass
      - ✓ Powder like residue can be stored for years
      - ✓ Organism revived by hydration and suitable liquid nutrient medium

F. Growth of Bacterial Cultures
- Refers to bacterial **growth in numbers, not size**
- **Bacterial division**
  - Normally reproduce by **binary fission** (most common method)
  - Few reproduce by **budding** (outgrowth that enlarges; becomes the size of parent, then separates)
  - A few filamentous species **fragment**
- **Generation time (GT)**
  - **The time required for a cell to divide and its population to double**
  - Varies among organism and their environment
  - **Most bacteria** have a GT of 1-3 hours; others need less time (mins) or more than 24 hours
- **Logarithmic representation of bacterial populations**
  - Calculates and graphs how bacterial division is a logarithmic progression
- **Phases of Growth**
  - Plotted by a **bacterial growth curve which shows growth of cells over time**
  - Consist of **four phases**
    - **Lag Phase**
      - ✓ **Little or no cell division;** can last one hour or several days; cells dormant; no increase in numbers
      - ✓ Synthesis of DNA, enzymes, and molecules
    - **Log (or Exponential Growth) Phase**
      - ✓ Cells dividing**; increasing in population;** most active metabolically**; sensitive phase**
    - **Stationary Phase**
      - ✓ Period of equilibrium; population stabilizes; **Growth rate slows** (nutrients used up, increase in waste); **dead cells = number of new cells**
    - **Death Phase**
      - ✓ Dead cells exceed new cells

G. Measurement of Microbial Growth by <u>Direct Methods</u>
- **Different methods used to measure cell growth**
  - **Plate Counts**
    - Most **frequently used method**
    - Measures number **of viable cells**
    - Takes time (24 hours or >) for visible colonies to form
    - Colonies often result from short segments of a chain or bacterial clump; reported as **colony-forming units (CFU)**

- **Serial dilution:** important to allow a limited number of colonies to develop in a plate (too many cause overcrowding and limit some cells from developing); original inoculum is diluted several times; ensure that some colony counts fall within the FDA "range" (plates with 25-250 colonies)
- **Done by either Pour Plate Method or Spread Plate Method**
  - ✓ **Pour Plate Method**
    - ❖ Colonies **grow in and on** solidified medium
  - ✓ **Spread Plate Method**
    - ❖ Inoculum **spread uniformly** over surface
- **Filtration**
  - Dealing with small quantity of bacteria (in lakes, streams)
  - Pass 100 ml H_2O thru a thin membrane filter with very small pores; bacteria stay behind
  - Bacteria then placed on petri dish with nutrients
    - ✓ Coliform bacteria (fecal contamination)
- **Most probable number (MPN) Method**
  - **Statistical estimating method**
- **Direct Microscopic Count**
  - A measured volume of bacteria is suspended in a liquid placed inside a designated area of a microscopic slide
  - Often used to count the number of bacteria in milk
  - Specially designed slide called a **Petroff-Hausser cell counter** also used
  - Motile bacteria difficult to count; dead cells likely to be counted as living cells
  - Need high volume microbial population to be countable

H. Estimating Bacterial Numbers by <u>Indirect Methods</u>
- Microbial numbers and activities measured by indirect methods
  - **Turbidity**
    - Bacteria multiply in a liquid medium; **medium becomes turbid or cloudy with cells**
    - Cloudiness of a liquid or loss of transparency because of insoluble matter
    - Instrument used: **Spectrophotometer (or colorimeter)**
      - ✓ A beam of light is transmitted through the bacteria (which is suspended in the liquid medium) to a light sensitive detector
      - ✓ Change in light will register on the instruments scale as **percentage of transmission; less light, more bacteria**
      - ✓ Absorbance (sometimes called Optical Density (OD)): a logarithmic expression used to plot growth
  - **Metabolic Activity**
    - Using metabolic waste products (CO_2 or acid) are directly proportional to the number of bacteria present
  - **Dry Weight**
    - **For filamentous bacteria and molds**
    - Bacteria and fungi: removed from their growth medium; filtered; dried; weighed

MICROBIOLOGY

CONTROL OF MICROBIAL GROWTH

A. Terms Related to Microbial Control
- **Sterilization**
  - **The destruction or removal of ALL living microorganisms**
    - **Heating** most common method used
  - Sterilizing agent used called a **sterilant**
  - Usually done by
    - **Steam under pressure, sterilizing gas (ethylene oxide), incineration, filtration**
- **Commercial Sterilization**
  - Heat treatment **to kill endospores in canned foods** (*Clostridium botulinum*)
- **Disinfection**
  - Destruction of **vegetative (non-endospore-forming)** pathogens on ***nonliving tissue***
  - Use chemicals (disinfectants) or physical agents
    - **Phenols, alcohols, aldehydes, surfactants, UV light, boiling water**
- **Antisepsis**
  - Destruction of **vegetative (non-endospore-forming)** pathogens on ***living tissue***
  - Chemicals used (**iodine, alcohol**)) called antiseptics
- **Degerming**
  - **Mechanical removal** of a limited area
  - Alcohol swabs
- **Sanitization**
  - **Lowers** the number of microorganisms on objects (eating and drinking utensils) **to safe public health levels;** minimize chance of disease transmission
  - Usually done by high temperature washing or dipping in a chemical disinfectant
- **Biocide (or Germicide): kills microorganisms** (certain exceptions, like endospores)
  - Bacteriocide: kills bacteria
  - Sporicide: kills endospores
  - Fungicide: kills fungi
  - Virucide: inactivates viruses
  - Algicide: kills algae
- **Bacteriostasis**
  - **Inhibit's growth and multiplication**
- **Sepsis (decay or putrid)**
  - Indicates bacterial contamination
  - **Aseptic: absence of significant contamination**

B. Rate of Microbial Death
- Microbial death is the permanent loss of a microorganisms ability to reproduce under normal environmental conditions
- Microbial death rate is a technique used to evaluate an antimicrobial agent
- Microbes, when treated with antimicrobial chemical or heat, die at constant rate
- The "effectiveness" of an antimicrobial agent is influenced by the number of "still present" microbes
- Factors influencing the effectiveness of antimicrobial treatments

- o **Environment**
  - Environmental influences: organic matter (in blood, feces, saliva) inhibit the action of chemical antimicrobials
- o **Time of Exposure**
  - Many antimicrobial agents need longer exposure to be effective
- o **Number of Microbes**
  - The more there are, the longer it takes to eliminate the entire population
- o **Microbial Characteristics**
  - Endospores, capsule, toxins

C. Actions of Microbial Control Agents
- Target of many microbial agents is **cell wall or plasma membrane**
- Damage causes cellular contents to leak into surrounding medium
- **Damage to Proteins and Nucleic Acids**
  - o Proteins: breaking (due to heat, chemicals) of hydrogen and covalent bonds results in **denaturation**
  - o Nucleic Acids (DNA and RNA): damage by heat, radiation, chemicals; all causes inability of cell to replicate or carry out normal metabolic functions

D. Physical Methods of Microbial Control
- When selecting methods, one must consider: what else is affected; economic considerations
- **Heat**
  - o **Temperature and Time** two important factors
  - o Kills by **denaturing the enzymes;** results in a three-dimensional change in shape→ **inactivation**
  - o Heat **resistance varies** among different microorganisms; expressed through three concepts
    - **Thermal death point (TDP): lowest temperature** in which all microbes in a particular liquid suspension are killed in 10 minutes
    - **Thermal death time (TDT): minimal length of time** for all microbes in a particular liquid suspension to be killed at a given temperature
    - **Decimal reduction time (DRT or D value): time in minutes** in which **90%** of the population of bacteria at a given time will be killed
  - o **Moist Heat Sterilization**
    - Kills by denaturation
    - **Boiling:** kills vegetative forms of bacterial pathogens, almost all viruses, fungi and their spores within **10 mins > at 100° C; endospores and some viruses** need longer times
    - **Steam under pressure:** requires temperatures above that of boiling water, under pressure
      - ✓ **Autoclaves:** preferred method of sterilization unless material can be damaged by heat or moisture **(culture media, instruments, IV equipment)**; at pressure of about 15 psi (120 ° C) method will kill **all** organisms **(not prions)** and their endospores in about 15-20 minutes
      - ✓ Sterilization indicators: commercially available methods to indicate if heat treatment has achieved sterilization (color strips, color indicators, specified bacterial endospores)
    - **Pasteurization:** mild heating; **sufficient to kill pathogenic organisms that cause spoilage** without affecting taste **(milk, yogurt, ice cream,..)**; lowers microbial numbers; **thermoduric** (heat-resistant) **bacteria survive** pasteurization, but unlikely to cause disease
      - ✓ Phosphatase test: enzyme naturally in milk; if product pasteurized, enzyme inactivated
      - ✓ Most milk pasteurization uses temperatures at 72° C for 15 seconds
        - ❖ Known as **high temperature short-time (HTST) pasteurization**
        - ❖ Milk **sterilized by ultra-high-temperature (UHT) treatments; used in places without refrigeration**

- o **Dry Heat Sterilization**
    - ■ Kills by oxidation effects
    - ■ Direct **flaming**: simplest method used
        - ✓ Heat the inoculating loop under a flame until the **wire turns to a red glow**
        - ✓ **Incineration** has same principle; sterilize and dispose
    - ■ **Hot-air sterilization**: items are placed in an oven at 170 ° C for 2 hours
- ● **Filtration**
    - o The **passage** of a liquid or gas through a **"screen" with pores** small enough to retain the microorganisms; may have a vacumn
    - o Used to sterilize "heat sensitive" material (culture media, vaccines, enzymes...)
    - o **HEPA (high-efficiency particulate air filters)** for operating rooms occupied by burn victims
    - o **Membrane filters**: made of plastic polymers or cellulose esters; for industrial and laboratory use; same principle as **HEPA**
- ● **Low Temperatures**
    - o **Refrigeration (0 °C to 7 °C):** reduces metabolic rate of most microbes to reduce spore formation; **bacteriostatic effect**
    - o **Freezing (-2 °C or lower):** renders microbes dormant, not necessarily kill them
- ● **High Pressure**
    - o Applied to liquid suspensions; pressure is transferred quickly and evenly
    - o **Alters the molecular structure of proteins and carbohydrates** leading to inactivation of vegetative bacterial cells
    - o Endospores relatively resistant
    - o Preserves flavor, color, and nutritional values of products
- ● **Desiccation**
    - o The **absence of H_2O;** organism is **unable to grow or reproduce,** but is **viable**
    - o Water added, resume growth and division
    - o **Lyophilization (freeze-drying):** a dehydration process where one freezes the material and then reducing the surrounding pressure to allow the frozen water to sublimate
    - o Viruses and bacterial endospores generally resistant
- ● **Osmotic Pressure**
    - o Using **high [ ]'s of salts and sugars** creates a **hypertonic environment** causing water to leave the cell
    - o Used in preserving foods (cured meats, preserves, jams)
    - o Molds and yeast much more capable to survive than bacteria
- ● **Radiation**
    - o Has various effects of cells, depending on its wavelength, intensity, and duration
        - ■ **Ionizing radiation**
            - ✓ Gamma rays, X-rays, high energy electron beams
            - ✓ Wavelength **shorter** than nonionizing radiation
            - ✓ **Destroys DNA**
            - ✓ Ionized particles "hit" vital portions of the cell; these "hits" cause **mutations to kill the microbe**
            - ✓ Used in the food industry, dental, and medical supplies (plastic syringes, surgical gloves, suture material)
        - ■ **Nonionizing radiation**
            - ✓ Wavelength **longer** than ionizing radiation
            - ✓ **UV light damages the DNA** of exposed cells; inhibits replication of DNA
            - ✓ Forms **thymine dimers**
            - ✓ In germicidal lamps (hospitals, nurseries, OR, cafeteria)

- **Microwaves**
  - ✓ Not much direct affect on microbes

E. Chemical Methods of Microbial Control
- Used to control growth of microbes **in living tissue and inanimate objects**
- Most reduce microbial populations to safe levels
- **Principles of Effective Disinfection**
  - o What organisms disinfectant will be effective against
  - o Concentration of the disinfectant affects its actions (dilute as follows)
  - o What is the nature of the material being disinfected (may interfere with the action of the disinfectant)
  - o pH of the medium
  - o Disinfectant should come in contact with microbes
  - o Left on surface for extended time
- **Evaluating a Disinfectant**
  - o Need to evaluate the effectiveness of the disinfectants and antiseptics
    - **Dilution Tests:** bacterial survival in recommended dilution of a disinfectant is determined
      - ✓ Dried cultures placed in a solution of disinfectant at a recommended concentration; left for a period of time at a certain temperature; then placed in a medium which allows growth
      - ✓ Effectiveness of disinfectant determined by the **number of cultures growing**
      - ✓ Also used for testing antimicrobial agents against: endospores, mycobacteria, fungi, viruses
    - **Disk-diffusion Method**
      - ✓ Disc of filtered paper soaked in a disinfectant; placed on inoculated medium
      - ✓ Effectiveness identified by a **zone of inhibition**
- **Types of Disinfectants**
  - o **Phenols and Phenolics**
    - **Phenols**
      - ✓ Derived from carbolic acid
      - ✓ **Disrupts plasma membrane** by denaturing proteins
      - ✓ Used to control surgical infections in the O.R.; control sewage odor
      - ✓ Used in lozenges
      - ✓ **Seldom used** as an antiseptic or disinfectant due **to irritation of skin and odor**
    - **Phenolics**
      - ✓ Derivatives of phenol (molecule chemically altered)
      - ✓ **Injures lipid containing plasma membranes** (mycobacterium)
      - ✓ Not as irritating; used on skin surfaces
      - ✓ **Lysol**
  - o **Bisphenols**
    - Derivative of phenol (two phenolic groups connected by a bridge)
    - **Disrupts plasma membrane**
    - Examples
      - ✓ **Hexachlorophene**
        - ❖ Ingredient in **pHisoHex**
          *Used during surgical and hospital microbial control procedures
          ***Gram positive staphylococci and streptococci susceptible**
          *Used in **nurseries: excessive use can cause neurological damage**
      - ✓ **Tricolsan**
        - ❖ In antibacterial soaps, tooth paste, kitchen cutting boards

- ❖ **Inhibits enzyme needed for biosynthesis of FA's (lipids)** which affect plasma membrane
- ❖ **Effective against gram positive (+) bacteria, certain gram negative (-) bacteria and yeast**

- o **Biguanides**
  - ■ Broad spectrum of activity
  - ■ Primarily affects **bacterial cell membranes** and some **enveloped viruses**
  - ■ Example
    - ✓ **Chlorhexidine**
      - ❖ Controls microbes on **skin and mucous membranes**
      - ❖ Contact with eye can cause damage
      - ❖ In surgical hand scrubs
      - ❖ **Effective against most gram positive (+) and gram negative (-) bacteria; yeasts**
    - ✓ **Alexidine**: more rapid in its action than chlorhexidine
- o **Halogens**
  - ■ **Nonmetallic chemical elements**
  - ■ Examples
    - ✓ **Iodine**
      - ❖ One of the oldest and most effective **antiseptics**
      - ❖ **Impairs protein synthesis and alters cell membranes**
      - ❖ **Effective against bacteria, many endospores, certain fungi, some viruses**
      - ❖ Available as **a tincture** (in solution with aqueous alcohol)
      - ❖ **Iodophor** (Iodine and an organic molecule): **less irritating; does not stain**
      - ❖ **Bentadine** and **isodine** both commercial preparations
    - ✓ **Chlorine**
      - ❖ Disinfectant in gas form or in combination with other chemicals
      - ❖ When added to H_2O forms **hypochlorous acid** (HOCl)
      - ❖ HOCl strong **oxidizing agent preventing cellular enzyme system** from functioning
      - ❖ Liquid form of gas used to disinfect municipal drinking H_2O, swimming pools, sewage
      - ❖ **Calcium hypochlorite** [$Ca(OCl)_2$]:disinfects dairy equipment; restaurant eating utensils
      - ❖ **Sodium hypochlorite:** used as a **disinfectant and bleach (Clorox)**
      - ❖ **Chlorine dioxide solution:** does not leave residual tastes or odors
      - ❖ **Chloramines:** combination of **chlorine and ammonia;** used in water treatment systems
- o **Alcohols**
  - ■ **Denature proteins** and **dissolve lipids**
  - ■ **Effective against bacteria and fungi**
  - ■ **Not effective against endospores or nonenveloped viruses**
  - ■ Examples
    - ✓ **Isopropanol (rubbing alcohol)**
    - ✓ **Ethanol (drinking)**
    - ✓ Alcohol-based hand sanitizers
- o **Heavy Metals**
  - ■ Several; can be **biocidal or antiseptic**
  - ■ **Denature enzymes**
  - ■ **Silver, mercury, copper, zinc:** small amounts have **"oligodynamic action"**

- ✓ **Silver**
  - ❖ **1% silver nitrate solution**: used as an antiseptic; used in past for ophthalmia neonatorum
  - ❖ Infused in plastic food containers, athletic shirts, and socks
  - ❖ **Silver sulfadiazine**: topical cream on burns
  - ❖ **Surfacine**: silver iodine
- ✓ **Mercury**
  - ❖ **Mercuric chloride**: used as a disinfectant; primarily a bacteriostatic; **toxic**
- ✓ **Copper**
  - ❖ **Copper sulfate**: used as an algicide (for reservoirs, ponds, swimming pools, fish tanks)
  - ❖ **Copper 8-hydroxyquinoline**: paints, fungal diseases of plants
  - ❖ **Xgel**: hand sanitizer
- ✓ **Zinc**
  - ❖ **Zinc chloride**: mouth wash
  - ❖ **Zinc pyrithione**: antidandruff shampoos

- o **Surface-active Agents (aka Surfactants)**
  - ■ **Decrease surface tension causing disruption of cell membranes**
    - ✓ **Soaps and Detergents**
      - ❖ Limited germicidal activity; important in **mechanical removal of microbes**
    - ✓ **Acid-Anionic Detergents**
      - ❖ Negatively charged part of the molecule **reacts with plasma membrane**
      - ❖ Nontoxic, noncorrosive, fast acting
      - ❖ Used in dairy and food-processing industries
- o **Quaternary Ammonium Compounds (Quats)**
  - ■ **The most widely used surface-active agents**
  - ■ Cleaning ability due to the positively charged portion of the molecule
  - ■ **Enzyme inhibition, protein denaturation, disrupt membranes**
  - ■ Strongly bactericidal against gram positive (+) bacteria
  - ■ Fungicidal, amoebicidal, virucidal
  - ■ Aseptic for skin, instruments, utensils
  - ■ Examples
    - ✓ **Zephiran** (benalkonium chloride)
    - ✓ **Cepacol** (cetylpyridinium chloride)
    - ✓ **Both:** antimicrobial, colorless, odorless, tasteless, nontoxic, stable, **except at high []'s**
  - ■ Certain species of *Pseudomonas* thrive and survive in **Quats**
- o **Chemical Food Preservatives**
  - ■ Added to foods to retard spoilage
  - ■ **Sulfur dioxide (SO_2):** used as a disinfectant in wine making
  - ■ **Sorbic acid** (potassium sorbate and sodium benzoate): **prevents mold** (cheese, soft drinks)
  - ■ **Calcium propionate: a fungistat** (used in bread)
  - ■ **Sodium nitrate and sodium nitrite**
    - ✓ **Prevent germination and growth of any botulism endospores**
    - ✓ Preserves the "red color" of meat products (ham, bacon, hot dogs, sausages)
    - ✓ Concern of nitrites with amino acids forming **nitrosamines (? Carcinogen)**
- o **Antibiotics**
  - ■ **Use is highly restricted**; certain ones used in food preservation
  - ■ Examples
    - ✓ Nisin: added to cheese, dairy products; inhibits growth of certain endospore-forming spoilage bacteria; a **bacteriocin;** tasteless, nontoxic, digestible

- ✓ **Natamycin: antifungal;** cheese
- ✓ Neither of clinical value
- o **Aldehydes**
  - ■ Among the most effective antimicrobials
  - ■ **Inactivate proteins** by forming covalent cross-links with several organic functional groups on proteins
  - ■ Examples
    - ✓ **Formaldehyde gas**
      - ❖ Excellent disinfectant
      - ❖ Available as **Formalin** (37% aqueous solution of the gas)
      - ❖ Used to **preserve biological specimens;** inactivate bacteria and viruses in vaccines
    - ✓ **Glutaraldehyde**
      - ❖ Less irritating and more effective than formaldehyde
      - ❖ Disinfects hospital instruments (respiratory therapy equipment)
      - ❖ In 2% solution **(Cidex)**
        *Bactericidal, tuberculocidal, virucidal in 10 minutes
        *Sporicidal in 3-10 hours
  - ■ Both **formaldehyde and glutaraldehyde** used by morticians **for embalming**
  - ■ **Ortho-phthalaldehyde (OPA):** possible replacement for glutaraldehyde; less irritating
- o **Chemical Sterilization**
  - ■ Gaseous chemosterilants frequently used as substitutes for physical sterilization procedures
  - ■ Requires a closed chamber
  - ■ Example
    - ✓ **Ethylene oxide**
      - ❖ **Gas**
      - ❖ Action depends on **alkylation;** leads to cross-linking of nucleic acids and proteins inhibiting vital cellular functions
      - ❖ **Kills all microbes and endospores**
      - ❖ Requires lengthy exposure time; toxic; explosive
    - ✓ **Chlorine dioxide**
      - ❖ Short-lived **gas**
      - ❖ Used in fumigation of closed buildings contaminated with endospores of anthrax
      - ❖ Used in water treatment to remove or reduce formation of certain carcinogenic compounds
- o **Plasma Sterilization**
  - ■ Possibly a **"fourth state of matter"** which a gas is excited producing **free radicals** to sterilize metal or plastic surgical instruments
  - ■ Requires low temperatures but expensive
- o **Supercritical Fluids**
  - ■ Combines chemical and physical methods
  - ■ Molecules **compressed** into a state of **both a liquid and gas**; organisms exposed are inactivated
  - ■ Example
    - ✓ **Carbon dioxide:** used to decontaminate medical implants (bone, tendons, ligaments)
- o **Peroxygens**
  - ■ Group of **oxidizing agents**
  - ■ Antimicrobial activity by **oxidizing molecules within the microbes, preventing metabolism**
  - ■ Examples

43

  ✓ **Ozone**: supplements chlorine to help neutralize taste and odors
  ✓ **Hydrogen peroxide**: disinfects **inanimate objects well**; heated, can be used as a sterilant
  ✓ **Benzoyl peroxide: acne**
  ✓ **Peracetic acid (peroxyactic acid or PAA): sterilant;** kills endospores and viruses within 30 mins; also used in disinfection of food-processing techniques

F. Microbial Characteristics and Microbial Control
  - **Many biocides are more effective against gram positive (+) bacteria, than gram negative (-)**
  - Principle factor in resistance is the **external LPS layer of gram negative (-) bacteria and porins**
  - **Cell wall** of some bacteria **has waxy, lipid-rich component** *(Mycobacterium tuberculosis)*
  - **Certain viruses** are resistant due to having **envelops**
  - **Bacterial endospores** affected by few biocides
  - **Prions** resistant to disinfectants and autoclaving

MICROBIOLOGY

MICROBIAL GENETICS

A. Genetics
- A branch of science which **studies heredity and how "traits"** (expressed characteristics) **are passed from one generation to the next**
- A **"trait"** is like an **"instruction"**; tells an organism how to do something (Ex: how to form a finger)
- Each **"instruction"** is contained in a **"gene"**
- There are **thousands of genes** necessary for an organism to grow
- **Genome is the genetic information in a cell;** organized into **chromosomes**
- **Chromosomes** are structures **containing DNA that carry the hereditary information**
- **Genomics is the sequencing and molecular characterization of genomes**
- **Genes are segments (sections) of DNA or RNA** placed in a specific sequence that "code" for a function
- **Genetic code: like "the set of rules" that determine how a nucleotide sequence is converted into the amino acid sequence of a protein**

B. Genotype and Phenotype
- **Genotype:** the **organisms DNA (collection of genes)**
- **Phenotype:** the actual, expressed properties; **the manifestation of genotype**
- Most of the cell's properties are from the **structures and functions of its proteins**
- **Most proteins** in microbes are either **enzymatic or structural**

C. DNA and Chromosomes
- Bacteria have **a single circular chromosome** consisting of **a single circular molecule of DNA** with **associated proteins**
- **The chromosome is looped and attached to one or more parts of the plasma membrane**
- **DNA is super coiled by enzymes** (topoisomerase II or DNA gyrase)
- The **entire genome** does not consist of back-to-back genes
- There are **noncoding regions** called **short tandem repeats (SRTs)**; these are repeating sequences of two to five base sequences; used in **DNA fingerprinting**
- Computers used to search for open-reading frames (regions of DNA likely to encode a protein)
- Sequencing and molecular characteristics of genomes called genomics

D. The Flow of Genetic Information
- **DNA replication** makes the flow of **genetic information from one generation to the next, possible**
  - **DNA replication occurs before cell division**
  - Each daughter receives a chromosome identical to the parent
  - **Genetic information is <u>also</u> transcribed into mRNA and then translated into a protein**

E. DNA Replication
- **One parent double stranded DNA molecule is unzipped and two identical daughter molecules made**
  - Replication begins when the parent ds DNA molecule unwinds
  - **Topoisomerase or gyrase** relaxes supercoiling

- o The two strands of parental DNA unwind by **helicase**
- o Free nucleotides in the cytoplasm match up to exposed bases of the single-stranded parental DNA
- o Newly added nucleotide is joined to the growing DNA strand by **DNA polymerase**
- o **DNA polymerase** also **proof reads** the new DNA strand; removes bases that do not match
- o DNA parental strand unwinds further allowing the addition of the next nucleotides
- o The **point** at which **replication occurs** called **replication fork**
- o As replication fork moves along parental DNA, **each unwound single strand combines with new nucleotides**
- o The **original and newly synthesized daughter strand rewind**
- o Now, **each new double-stranded DNA molecule contains one original (conserved) and one new strand**; referred to as **semiconservative replication**

- ● **Structure of DNA**
  - o The **paired DNA strands** are oriented in opposite directions, relative to each other
  - o The carbon atoms of the sugar component of each nucleotide are numbered 1' to 5'
  - o The end with the hydroxyl attached to the 3' carbon called 3' end of DNA
  - o The end having a phosphate attached to the 5' carbon called 5' end of DNA
  - o Two strands fit together dictating that the 5'→3' direction of one strands runs counter to the 5'→3' of the other strand
  - o DNA replication requires energy
  - o DNA replication in some bacteria occurs **bidirectionally** around the chromosome
    - ■ **Two replication forks move in opposite directions;** eventually meet when replication is done
    - ■ The two loops are separated by a **topoisomerase**
  - o **DNA is synthesized in <u>one</u> direction : 5'→3'**
    - ■ **Leading strand**: synthesized continually by DNA polymerase
    - ■ **Lagging strand**: synthesized discontinually
      - ✓ **Primase** (an **RNA polymerase**) synthesizes a short **RNA primer to start synthesis**
      - ✓ **DNA polymerase** digests **the primer;** replaces it with new DNA fragments **(Okazaki fragments)**
      - ✓ **DNA ligase** joins the newly made DNA fragments

F. RNA and Protein Synthesis (in Bacterial Cells)

- ● **The process in which information in DNA is used to make proteins**
- ● Process consist of
  - o **Transcription**: genetic information in DNA is copied into a complementary base sequence of RNA
  - o **Translation**: information encoded in RNA is synthesized to specific proteins
- ● Requires **RNA** (nucleotides with bases A, C, G, U)
- ● Three types of RNA involved in protein synthesis
  - o **Ribosomal RNA (rRNA):** the enzymatic part of ribosomes
  - o **Transfer RNA (tRNA):** transports amino acids to the ribosomes in order to synthesize proteins
  - o **Messenger RNA (mRNA):** carries the genetic information from the DNA into the cytoplasm to ribosomes where the proteins are made
- ● **RNA polymerase** synthesizes **rRNA, tRNA, mRNA**

G. Protein Synthesis

- ● Includes **transcription, RNA processing, and translation**
- ● **Transcription**
  - o The synthesis of **a complimentary strand of RNA from a DNA template**
    - ■ A strand of **mRNA** is synthesized using a specific portion of cell's **DNA** as a template

- ■ The genetic information stored in DNA is **rewritten** so the information appears in the base sequence of **mRNA**
  - o Requires **RNA polymerase** and **RNA nucleotides**
  - o Begins when RNA polymerase binds to DNA at a **promoter site** (RNA synthesized in the 5'→3' direction)
  - o DNA unwinds
  - o **RNA polymerase** assembles free nucleotides with nucleotide bases on the DNA template strand
  - o **RNA polymerase** moves along the DNA as the new RNA strand grows
  - o **RNA polymerase** reaches a **terminator site** on the DNA and is stopped
  - o The new single stranded RNA and the RNA polymerase are released
  - o **mRNA**, acting as an intermediate, **carries the coded information** (for making specific proteins from DNA) **to ribosomes**
  - o Once transcription is completed, the information of the mRNA is turned into a protein
- ● **Translation**
  - o Process in which the **genetic information** (encoded in mRNA) **is translated into a specific sequence of amino acids (aa's) that produce proteins**
    - ■ Components needed to begin translation: two **ribosomal subunits, a tRNA with the anticodon UAC, mRNA, protein factors);** components all come together to start translation
  - o **The language of mRNA is in the form of codons (**groups of three nucleotides, such as AUG, GGC, AAA)
  - o There are **64 codons:** 61 are sense codons, 3 are nonsense codons
    - ■ **Sense codons:** code for amino acids
    - ■ **Nonsense codons (or stop codons):** do not code for aa's; **signal the end of protein synthesis**
  - o **Start codon: AUG**
  - o **Stop codons: UAA, UAG, UGA**
  - o Each **codon** 'codes' for **a particular amino acid** that will be in the protein
  - o **Codons** are written in terms of their base sequence in **mRNA**
  - o The **genetic code is degenerate**
    - ■ There are **64** possible **codons,** but **only 20 amino acids**
    - ■ Most amino acids are coded for by more than one codon; this allows a certain amount of change, or mutation, in the DNA without affecting the protein produced
  - o The **aa** sequences are brought to the translation site in the ribosomes and assembled into a chain
  - o **tRNA** recognizes specific codons
  - o Each **tRNA has an anticodon** which is **complementary to the bases on the codon**
  - o These bases **(codon and anticodon)** are paired and the amino acids are brought to the chain; this **produces a polypeptide**
  - o The proper **aa's** are brought into line, one by one, producing a **polypeptide chain**
  - o **Translation ends** when a **nonsense code is reached**
    - ■ The ribosome comes apart; the mRNA and polypeptide chain are released
    - ■ The ribosome, mRNA, and tRNA are available to be used again
- ● **In Prokaryotic cells**
  - o **Translation** of mRNA into proteins **can begin before transcription is complete**
- ● **In Eukaryotic cells**
  - o **Transcription** takes place in the nucleus
  - o **RNA** undergoes processing before leaving the nucleus
  - o Have regions of genes **(exons)** that code for proteins interrupted by **noncoding DNA (introns)**
  - o **RNA polymerase** synthesizes an **RNA transcript** containing copies of **introns**
  - o **small nuclear ribonucleoproteins (snRNPs)** remove the **introns** and **join the exons together**

H. Regulation of Bacterial Gene Expression
- All metabolic reactions are catalyzed by enzymes
- **There are mechanisms which prevents cells from performing unneeded chemical reactions**
- These mechanisms **prevent synthesis of enzymes** that are not needed, **or regulate the production of enzymes** so they are present only when needed
- Cells save energy by making only those proteins needed
- Many genes are **constitutive (unregulated):** their **products are constantly produced at a fixed rate**
  - Example: glycolysis
- **Pre-transcriptional Control**
  - Two mechanisms known to regulate the **transcription of mRNA**
    - **Repression**
      - ✓ **Inhibits** gene expression by regulatory proteins called **repressors**
      - ✓ Decreasing synthesis of enzymes
      - ✓ Blocks **RNA polymerase to initiate transcription**
      - ✓ Default position of a **repressor gene** is <u>*on*</u>
    - **Induction**
      - ✓ **Activates** transcription **of a gene or genes**
      - ✓ A *substance* that induces transcription called **an inducer**
      - ✓ The **enzymes synthesized** in the presence of **inducers** called *inducible enzymes*
      - ✓ Example: *E. coli*
        - ❖ Genes needed for **lactose metabolism in** *E. coli*
          *One codes for **β-galactosidase** (splits substrate lactose into glucose and galactose)
          *In the **absence of lactose,** organism contains almost **no β-galactosidase**
          *In the **presense of lactose,** β-galatosidase **produced** in large quantities
          *Lactose in cell converted to **allolactose** (the **inducer** for these genes)
      - ✓ Default position of **an inducible gene** is <u>*off*</u>
  - These two mechanisms **control formation and amounts of enzymes** in cell, **not the activities of the enzyme**
  - **The Operon Model of Gene Expression**
    - Describes the control of gene expression by induction and repression
    - Model based on **lactose catabolism in** *E. coli*
    - Enzymes involved are
      - ✓ **β-galactosidase:** splits **lactose** into **glucose and galactose**
      - ✓ **Lac permease:** transports lactose into cell
      - ✓ **Transacetylase:** metabolizes certain disaccharides other than lactose
    - The **genes for these enzymes** are next to each other on the bacterial chromosome
    - These genes are called **structural genes** which are next to a **control region** on the DNA
    - When **lactose** is added to the culture medium, the **lac structural genes** are quickly transcribed and translated
      - ✓ Control region of the **lac operon** contain **two short segments** of DNA
        - ❖ **Promoter:** region of DNA where **RNA polymerase** initates **transcription**
        - ❖ **Operator:** acts as a **go or stop** signal for transcription of the structural genes
    - **Operon**
      - ✓ Consists of the **promoter (P) site,** the **operator (O) site,** and **the structural genes** which code for the protein
      - ✓ A **regulatory gene (the I gene)** encodes a **repressor protein** which switches **inducible and repressor operons** <u>on</u> or <u>off</u>
      - ✓ <u>Inducible operon:</u> the **lac operon**

- ❖ In the **absence of lactose, repressor** binds to **operator (O) site,** preventing transcription
- ❖ If **lactose present, repressor** binds to a **metabolite of lactose; enzymes** to digest lactose **transcribed**
  - ✓ <u>Repressible operon</u>: the **trp (tryptophan) operon**
    - ❖ **The structural genes are transcribed until they are repressed (or turned off)**
      *The **structural genes** are transcribed and translated, leading to **tryptophan synthesis**
      *When **excess tryptophan** present, **tryptophan acts as a corepressor; binds to** the **repressor protein**
      *The **repressor protein** now can bind to the **operator (O)** site, **stopping tryptophan synthesis**
- o **Positive Regulation**
  - ■ Regulation of the **lac operon** also depends on level of **glucose** in the medium
  - ■ When glucose is no longer available (a form of stress to the cell), **cAMP** (derived from **ATP**) accumulates in the cell
  - ■ **cAMP** is an example of an **alarmone**: a chemical signal which promotes a cell's response to stress (environmental or nutritional)
  - ■ The **cAMP binds to** the allosteric site of catabolic activator protein **(CAP)**
  - ■ **CAP** binds to the **lac promoter;** this initiates transcription; makes it easier for **RNA polymerase** to bind to **promoter (P) site** and transcribe large amounts of **mRNA** for lactose digestion
  - ■ **Transcription** of the lac operon requires both the **presence of lactose and absence of glucose**
  - ■ Positive Regulation involving **cAMP** allows cells to grow on other sugars
    - ✓ Catabolic repression: inhibition of the metabolism of alternative carbon sources by glucose; when glucose is available, **cAMP** levels low; **CAP not bound**
- o **Epigenetic Control**
  - ■ Eukaryotes and bacterial cells **can turn genes off by methylating** certain nucleotides
  - ■ These **methylated (off) genes** are passed to offspring
  - ■ The **genes** can be turned **on** in a later generation
  - ■ Called **epigenetic inheritance**
- ● <u>Post-transcriptional Control</u>
  - o Some regulatory mechanisms **stop protein synthesis** <u>after</u> **transcription** has occurred
  - o **microRNAs (miRNAs):** ssRNA molecules which **inhibit protein production** in eukaryotic cells
  - o **miRNAs,** in humans, produced during development; allow different cells to produce different proteins
    - ■ Examples: heart and skin cells; both have same genes but produce different proteins
  - o In bacteria **miRNAs** help cope with environmental stresses
  - o An **miRNA** base-pairs with a **complementary mRNA** forming a **double-stranded (ds) RNA**
  - o This **ds RNA** is destroyed so the **mRNA-encoded protein is not made**

I. Mutations
- ● Are **permanent change** in the base sequence of DNA
- ● This "**change**" will cause a change in the product (**harmful or beneficial**)
- ● **Many** simple mutations are **silent (neutral);** the change causes **no change in the activity of the product**
  - o **Silent mutations** commonly occur when **one nucleotide** is **substituted for another**
  - o The resulting new codon might still code for the amino acid (aa)

- o Even if the aa is changed, the function of the protein may not change
- **Types of Mutations**
  - o **Point (or base substitution) mutation**
    - **Most common** type
    - **Single base** in the DNA sequence **replaced** with a **different base**
    - DNA replicates resulting in a **substituted base pair**
    - **No change in amino acid (aa) sequence**
  - o **Missense mutation**
    - Occurs when **point mutation** results in **an amino acid substitution**
    - Codes for a **different aa**
    - Example
      - ✓ **Sickle cell disease**; results in the change from **glutamic acid to valine**
  - o **Nonsense mutation**
    - A base substitution creating a **stop (premature termination** of transcription**) codon** which prevents the synthesis of a protein
  - o **Frameshift mutations**
    - One or a few nucleotide pairs are **deleted or inserted** in the DNA
    - Can causes changes in many amino acids downstream
    - Can result in altered amino acids and production of inactive proteins
  - o **Spontaneous mutations**
    - Naturally occurring; occur in the **absence of mutagen** causing agents
  - o **Induced mutations**
    - Occurs in the laboratory

J. Mutagens

- **Agents** in the environment which directly or indirectly **bring about mutations**
  - o **Chemical mutagens**
    - **Nitrous acid:** alters an **adenine (A)** where it pairs with **cytosine (C) instead of thymine (T)**
    - **Nucleoside analogues:** similar to normal nitrogenous bases, **but** have altered base-pairing properties; some antiviral and antitumor drugs
    - **Frame shift mutagens:** benzopyrene (in smoke and soot); aflatoxin (produced by mold)
  - o **Radiation**
    - **Xrays, gamma rays**
      - ✓ **Ionize** atoms and molecules which damage DNA; cause electrons to pop out of their usual shells
    - **Ultraviolet (UV) light**
      - ✓ **Nonionizing** component of sunlight
      - ✓ **Forms harmful covalent bonds**; adjacent **thymines cross-link** to form **"thymine dimers"**
      - ✓ Bacteria and other organisms have **enzymes to repair the UV damage**
        - ❖ Photolyases (light-repair enzymes); nucleotide excision repair; methylases

K. Frequency of Mutations

- **Mutation rate** is the probability that a gene will mutate when the cell divides
- **Mutations** usually occur randomly along the chromosome
- Most **mutations** are harmful and likely to be removed when cell dies
- A few **mutations** are beneficial (antibiotic resistance for the bacteria)

L. Identifying Mutants

- Mutants can be detected by selecting or testing for an altered phenotype

- Experiments usually **performed with bacteria**
  - o Reproduce rapidly; have one copy of each gene/cell
- **Positive (direct) selection**
  - o Involves the **detection of mutant cells by the rejection of the unmutated parent cells**
    - ■ Example: Penicillin resistant bacteria
      - ✓ When bacterial cells are plated on a medium containing penicillin, the mutants (resistant) will grow; the normal will not grow
- **Negative (indirect) selection**
  - o Process **selects a cell that cannot perform a certain function;** using the **replica plating technique**
    - ■ Example: Bacteria that has lost their ability to synthesize histidine
      - ✓ About 100 **bacteria are inoculated** on an agar plate (**called master plate**) **containing** medium with **histidine** which cells can grow
      - ✓ Incubated; each cell reproduces forming a colony
      - ✓ **Pad of sterile material** (latex, velvet, filter paper) pressed over **master plate;** some cells adhere
      - ✓ The **Pad of sterile material,** then **pressed onto two or more sterile plates**
        - ❖ One plate contains **medium without histidine**
        - ❖ One plate contains **medium with histidine**
      - ✓ Colonies that grows on medium **with histidine,** but **cannot grow on medium without histidine** considered an **auxotroph**
        - ❖ **Auxotroph:** a mutant microbe that has a nutritional need that is absent in the parent
      - ✓ The **mutant colony** can be identified on the **master plate**
  - o **Replica plating** is effective in isolating mutants the require one or more growth factors

M. Identifying Chemical Carcinogens
- Many mutagens are found to be carcinogens (cause cancer)
- Testing procedures involve animals, and time consuming
- Now there are faster, less expensive tests for preliminary screen
  - o **Ames test**
    - ■ Uses bacteria as carcinogen indicators
    - ■ Based on the observation that **exposure of mutant bacteria to mutagenic substances may cause new mutations that will reverse the effect of the original mutation**
    - ■ Called **reversions**
    - ■ The test measures **the reversion of histidine auxotrophs** of *Salmonella* (his⁻ cells) to his⁺ **after treatment with a mutagen**
      - ✓ Bacteria incubated in both the presence and absence of the substance being tested
      - ✓ The chemical to be tested and the mutant bacteria are incubated together with rat liver extract (source of activation enzymes)
      - ✓ If substance is mutagenic, will cause reversion of his⁻ bacteria to his⁺ bacteria

N. Genetic Transfer and Recombination
- **Genetic Recombination**
  - o Is the **exchange of genes between two DNA molecules** to form new combinations of genes on a chromosome; contributes to genetic diversity
  - o If a cell picks up foreign DNA (donor DNA), some could insert into the cells chromosome; called **crossing over** ; two chromosomes "cross over", break, and rejoin, sometimes in several locations

- o With **crossing over**, the **DNA has recombined** so that the chromosome now carries a portion of donor's DNA
- o **Vertical gene transfer**
  - ■ Occurs during reproduction (genes passed from parent to offspring)
  - ■ Plants, animals
- o **Horizontal gene transfer**
  - ■ Passing genes laterally to other microbes of the same generation
  - ■ Involves a donor cell and a recipient cell
- **Transformation in Bacteria**
  - o Genes are transferred from one bacterium to another as **"naked" DNA** in solution
  - o **Griffith's experiment**
    - ■ **Living encapsulated** bacteria injected into mouse→**mouse dies**→colonies of encapsulated bacteria **isolated** from dead mouse
    - ■ **Living nonencapsulated** bacteria injected into mouse→**mouse lives**→**few colonies** of **nonencapsulated live** (destroyed by phagocytes)
    - ■ **Heat-killed encapsulated** bacteria injected into mouse→**mouse lives**→**no colonies**
    - ■ **Living nonencapsulated and heat-killed encapsulated** bacteria injected into mouse→**mouse dies**→**colonies of encapsulated bacteria grow**
  - o Bacterial transformation can be carried out without mice; can be done in broth
- **Conjugation in Bacteria**
  - o **Requires direct cell-to-cell contact**
  - o Mediated by a **plasmid** (circular piece of DNA that replicates independently from the cells chromosome)
  - o Conjugating cells must be either
    - ■ **Donor** cell: carries the **plasmid**
    - ■ **Recipient** cell: does not
  - o Example: *Escherichia coli*
    - ■ **F factor** (fertility factor): first plasmid observed to be transferred
    - ■ **Donor cell (F⁺):** carrying F factors; transfers plasmid to
    - ■ **Recipient cell (F⁻):** as a result, **become F⁺ cell**
  - o In some cells, the factor integrates **into the chromosome**, producing an **Hfr cell (high frequency of recombination)**
    - ■ During conjugation, an **Hfr cell** can transfer **chromosomal DNA** to an **F⁻ cell**
- **Transduction in Bacteria**
  - o Mechanism which bacterial DNA is transferred from a donor cell to a recipient cell **in a virus** which infects bacteria (called a **bacteriophage**)
  - o Two forms of **Transduction**
    - ■ **Generalized transduction: any** bacterial DNA can be transferred
    - ■ **Specialized transduction:** only **certain bacterial** genes are transferred
- **Plasmids and Transposons**
  - o Both are **genetic elements** that provide mechanisms for genetic change; In prokaryotes and eukaryotes
    - ■ **Plasmids**
      - ✓ **Self-replicating circular molecules of DNA** carrying genes that are not essential for the cells survival
      - ✓ **Several types**
        - ❖ Conjugative: F factor carries genes for sex pili and for transfer of the plasmid to another cell
        - ❖ Dissimilation: code for enzymes that trigger catabolism of unusual sugars and hydrocarbons

❖   Carrying genes for toxins or bacterocins: enhance pathogenicity

❖   Resistant factors: bacteria acquire resistance through spread of genes from one organism to another

- **Transposons**
  - ✓ Small segments of DNA that **can move** from one region of a DNA molecule to another; on the same chromosome or to a different chromosome or plasmid
  - ✓ Found in genetic material of viruses
  - ✓ **Types**
    - ❖ **Simple:** also called **insertion sequences (IS);** contain only a gene that codes for an enzyme (transposase: catalyzes the cutting and resealing of DNA that occurs in transposition) and recognition sites
    - ❖ **Complex:** carry **other genes** (for enterotoxins, antibiotic resistance,..) **not connected** with the transposition process

O. Genes and Evolution

- Genetic mutation and recombination provide diversity in the cells
- Provides evolution and natural selection

MICROBIOLOGY

BIOTECHNOLOGY AND DNA TECHNOLOGY

A. Introduction to Biotechnology
- **Biotechnology is the genetic alteration of an organism, cells, or cell components to make a product**
- Commercial production of foods, antibiotics, vaccines, vitamins, etc…
- **Inserting genes into cells** made possible by **recombinant DNA (rDNA) technology,** sometimes called **genetic engineering**
- **Recombinant DNA (rDNA) Technology**
  - A human gene can be inserted into the DNA of a bacterium, or a gene from a virus into a yeast
  - The recipient is made to express the gene, which will code for a commercially useful product
  - This technique can be used to make thousands of copies of the same DNA molecule
- **An Overview of Recombinant DNA Procedures**
  - The desired gene is inserted into a **DNA vector** (plasmid or viral genome)
  - The **vector** replicates independently
  - The recombinant vector DNA is taken up by a bacterium which can multiply
  - The bacterium containing the recombinant vector is grown in culture to form a **clone** (genetically identical cells)
  - One can isolate or **"harvest" large quantities** of the **gene of interest or** if the gene of interest is expressed in the cell clone, **its protein product** can be "harvested" and used

B. Tools of Biotechnology
- Bacteria and fungi from natural environments (soil, water) are isolated to **find the organisms that produce the desired product**
  - **Selection**
    - Organisms with features which **enhance survival more likely to survive and reproduce** (natural selection)
    - **Humans use artificial selection** (choosing one organism from a population to grow because of its desirable traits: **selected breeds of animals or strains of plants**)
  - **Mutation**
    - **Mutagens** can be used to **cause mutations which might result in a microbe with desirable traits** (Ex: Penicillium)
    - Site-directed mutagenesis is used to make a specific change in a gene (Ex: changing one amino acid to make a better soap)
  - **Restriction Enzymes**
    - DNA cutting enzymes in many bacteria
    - **Recognizes and cuts (digest) a particular nucleotide sequence in DNA**
    - **Restriction enzymes** used in cloning experiments recognize four-, six-, or eight-base sequences
    - Cuts produce DNA fragments with characteristic ends
      - ✓ **Blunt ends:** some enzymes cut both strands of DNA in **same place**
      - ✓ **Sticky ends:** staggered cuts in the two strands; cuts not directly opposite each other
        - ❖ Most useful in **rDNA**; can be used to join two **fragments of DNA** that were cut by same restriction enzyme

❖ Sticky ends stick to stretches of ssDNA by complementary base pairing
❖ Sticky ends join by hydrogen bonding
- **DNA ligase** covalently **links the DNA pieces,** producing an rDNA molecule

o **Vectors**
- **Self-replication is the most important property**
- Any DNA inserted in the vector will be replicated
- A type of vehicle for the replication of desired DNA sequences
- **Smaller vectors** easier to manipulate outside of cell during rDNA procedures
- **Plasmid** (circular DNA molecule which replicates without a chromosome) **or virus** used to insert genes into a cell
- Circular form important in protecting the vector from destruction by the recipient
- Some plasmids, called **shuttle vectors,** can exist in different species; used to move cloned DNA sequences among organisms
  ✓ Example: inserting herbicide resistance genes into plants
- **Viral DNA**
  ✓ Can usually accept larger pieces of foreign DNA than plasmids
  ✓ Once inside viral vector, it can be cloned in the virus's host cells
  ✓ Retroviruses, adenoviruses, herpesviruses used

o **Polymerase Chain Reaction (PCR)**
- Technique where **small specific sequences of DNA** can be **quickly amplified** (increased to quantities large enough for analysis)
  ✓ Each strand of the target DNA will serve as a template for DNA synthesis
  ✓ Added to this DNA are: the four nucleotides, enzyme for catalyzing the synthesis **(DNA polymerase), primers** (to start the reaction and hybridize to the fragments to be amplified)
  ✓ The **polymerase** synthesizes new complementary strands
  ✓ After each cycle, the DNA is heated to convert all the new DNA into single strands
  ✓ Each newly synthesized DNA strand serves as a template for more new DNA
- All necessary reagents added to a tube, and placed in a **thermal cycle**
- The amplified DNA seen by gel electrophoresis
- In **real-time PCR or quantitative PCR,** newly made DNA tagged with a fluorescent dye ; the levels of fluorescence can be measured after every cycle
- **Reverse-transcription PCR:** uses viral RNA or a cell's mRNA as a template; **reverse transcriptase** (an enzyme), makes DNA from the RNA template, and the DNA is amplified

C. Techniques of Genetic Modification
- **Inserting Foreign DNA into Cells**
  o DNA molecules need to be manipulated outside the cell and returned to living cells
  o Ways to introduce DNA into a cell
  - **Transformation:** cells take up **naked DNA;** chemical treatments used to make cells "competent"
  - **Electroporation:** current to produce pores in membranes of cells; DNA enters cells
  - **Protoplast fusion:** joining of cells whose cell walls have been removed (called **protoplast)**
  - **Gene gun:** shooting DNA-coated "bullets" into cells
  - **Microinjection:** micropipette punctures plasma membrane
- **Obtaining DNA**
  o **Two main sources of obtaining genes**
  - **Gene Libraries**
    ✓ Extracting the organisms DNA; cutting up the entire genome with restriction enzymes; inserting the fragments into plasmids or phages; produce collection of DNA clones

- ✓ Cloning from eukaryotic cells
  - ❖ Genes contain both **exons** (code for protein) and **introns** (do not code for protein)
  - ❖ Requires **reverse transcriptase** to synthesize **complementary DNA (cDNA)**
- ■ **Synthetic DNA**
  - ✓ Genes made in vitro with the aid of DNA synthesis machines
  - ✓ Short sequences of DNA can by synthesized
- ● **Selecting a Clone**
  - o In cloning it is necessary to **select a particular cell** which **contains the specific gene** of interest
  - o Typical screening procedure known as **blue-white screening**, from the color of the bacterial colonies formed at the end of the screening process
    - ■ Plasmid used has genes coding for ampicillin resistance (**ampR**) and a gene for the enzyme β-galactosidase (**lacZ**)
    - ■ Plasmid DNA and foreign (desired) DNA are cut with same restrictive enzyme
    - ■ Foreign (desired) DNA inserted into the plasmid (into the β-galactosidase gene site); this inactivates the lacZ gene; now we have a recombinant plasmid
    - ■ The recombinant plasmid is introduced into a bacterium; the bacterium becomes ampicillin-resistant
    - ■ The treated bacteria are spread on agar plate containing ampicillin and a β-galactosidase substrate (X-gal); incubated
      - ✓ **White colonies:** picked up the **recombinant plasmid;** clones are resistant to ampicillin and unable to hydrolyze X-gal
      - ✓ **Blue colonies: received original plasmid**; clones resistant to ampicillin and will hydrolyze X-gal producing galactose and an indigo compound making the colonies blue
      - ✓ Clones lacking the vector will not grow
  - o **Colony hybridization** is **a method used to identify cells that carry a specific cloned gene**
    - ■ DNA probes (short segments of ssDNA complementary to the desired gene) are synthesized
      - ✓ If DNA probe finds a match, will adhere to target gene
      - ✓ The DNA probe is labeled with radioactive element or fluorescent dye to help in identification
- ● **Making a Gene Product**
  - o *Escherichia coli* most often used to synthesize gene products; easily grown; genome is well know
  - o To obtain product, *Escherichia coli* must be lysed, or the gene inserted must be linked to a gene that produces a naturally secreted protein
  - o *Escherichia coli* (*E.* coli) has disadvantages: produces an **endotoxin** which can contaminate
  - o **Yeast** are used and likely to secrete a gene product
  - o **Mammalian cells** genetically modified can produce proteins such as hormones
  - o **Plant cells** can be used to produce plants with new and different properties

D. Applications of rDNA
- ● Cloned genes can produce useful substances more efficiently and cheaper
- ● Obtaining information from cloned DNA is useful in medicine, forensics, research
- ● Cloned genes can be used to alter characteristics of cells or organisms
  - o **Therapeutic Applications**
    - ■ Producing human insulin: *E. coli*
    - ■ Somatostatin: *E. coli*
    - ■ Subunit vaccines: use genetically modified yeast or viruses
    - ■ DNA vaccines: usually circular plasmids consisting of rDNA cloned in bacteria
    - ■ Human blood: genetically modified pigs
    - ■ Gene Therapy: providing cures for some genetic disorders: hemophilia B

        ✓ Gene silencing: a defense against viruses and transposons; silences the expression of a gene

        ✓ Technology called **RNA interference (RNAi)** offering promise for gene therapy, cancer treatment, viral infections

   o **Genome Projects**

      ■ The first genome sequenced was from a bacteriophage (1977)

      ■ *Haemophilus influenza* (1975)

      ■ 1000 prokaryotic and over 400 eukaryotic genomes have been sequenced

      ■ Shotgun sequencing: small pieces of genome sequenced and then assembled using a computer

      ■ **Metagenomics:** study of genetic material taken directly from environmental samples

   o **Scientific Applications**

      ■ Techniques used to increase the understanding of DNA, genetic fingerprinting, gene therapy

      ■ Once a large amount of DNA is available, different **analytic techniques** can be used to "read" the information in the DNA

         ✓ **Bioinformatics:** uses computer applications to study genetic data

         ✓ **Proteomics:** the science of determining all of the proteins expressed in a cell

         ✓ **Reverse genetics:** attempts to connect a given genetic sequence with specific effects on the organism

         ✓ **Southern blotting:** used to locate a gene in a cell

         ✓ **DNA probes:** can be used to identify a pathogen in body tissue or food

         ✓ **Forensic Microbiology:** uses **DNA fingerprinting** to help identify bacterial or viral pathogens

         ✓ **Nanotechnology:** the design and manufacture of extremely small electronic circuits and devices built at the molecular level of matter; researchers are using **bacteria to provide nanospheres** for drug targeting and delivery

   o **Agricultural Applications**

      ■ Cells from certain plants can be cloned to produce whole plants from which seeds can be harvested

      ■ Recombinant DNA can be introduced into plant cells several ways: protoplast fusion, DNA-coated bullets: **Ti plasmid**

      ■ Genes have been engineered into crop plants to enhance resistance

      ■ **Antisense DNA technology:** used to prevent expression of unwanted proteins

      ■ Genes genetically modified to enhance nitrogen fixation

      ■ Produce biological insecticides and certain growth hormones

E. Safety Issues and the Ethics of using rDNA

● **Strict safety standards are enforced to avoid accidental release of genetically altered microorganisms**

● Some microbes intended for use in the environment will contain suicide genes in order not to persist in the environment

● **Genetic testing for diseases**

   o Insurance companies and/or employers have access to persons genetic records

   o Certain people targeted for breeding or sterilization

   o Genetic counseling available to everyone

● **Are modified crops safe for consumption and release into environment?**

MICROBIOLOGY

CLASSIFICATION OF MICROORGANISMS

A. Taxonomy
- Is the science of classifying living forms
- Used to establish the relationships between one group of organisms and another, and differentiate between them

B. Phylogenetic Relationships
- The number of living organisms range from 10 to 100 million
- **Taxonomy** is used to show degrees of similarities among organisms
- **Phylogeny** is the study of the evolutionary history of organisms; shows relationships among organisms
- New techniques in molecular biology reveal there are **two types of prokaryotic cell and one type of eukaryotic cell**
- These **three cell types** based on differences in nucleotide sequencing in **ribosomal RNA (rRNA)**
- Living organisms are classified into **three domains** (based on **rRNA**, membrane lipid, structure, tRNA molecules, sensitivity to antibiotics)
  - **The Three Domains**
    - **Eukaryra:** animals, plants, fungus
    - **Bacteria: prokaryotes** with **peptidoglycan** in cell wall
    - **Archaea: prokaryotes without peptidoglycan** in their cell walls
  - Each domain shares genes with other domains
  - Endosymbiotic theory states eukaryotic cells evolved from prokaryotic cells living inside one another
- **Phylogenetic Hierarchy**
  - Groups organisms according to common properties; a group of organisms evolved from a common ancestor
  - **Each species retains some of the characteristics of their ancestors**
  - Information used in classifying and determining phylogenetic relationships comes **from fossils**
    - Available for **eukaryotes**
    - Not available for **most prokaryotes**

C. Classification of Organisms
- Organisms are grouped according to similar characteristics and assigned a **unique scientific name**
- **Scientific Nomenclature**
  - A system of scientific names developed
  - **Binomial nomenclature**
    - Every organism is assigned **two names**
      - ✓ **Genus:** always capitalized; always a noun
      - ✓ **Species (specific epithet): lower** case; usually an adjective
    - Both names printed underlined or italicized
      - ✓ Example: *Rhizopus stolonifer Rhizo-* (root); *stolo-* (shoot)
- **The Taxonomic Hierarchy**
  - Organisms are grouped into a series of subdivisions

- o Each group is more comprehensive
- o **Hierarchy**
  - ■ Species→Genus→Family→Order→Class→Phylum→Kingdom→Domain→All organisms
- o **Eukaryotic species are closely related organisms: breed amongst themselves**
- **Classification of Prokaryotes**
  - o Found in **Bergey's Manual of Systemic Bacteriology**
    - ■ Prokaryotes divided into two domains
      - ✓ **Bacteria**
      - ✓ **Archaea**
    - ■ Classification based on similarities on nucleotide sequences of **rRNA**
- **Classification of Eukaryotes**
  - o Classified into the Kingdom Fungi, Plantae, or Animalia
    - ■ **Kingdom Fungi:** absorb dissolved organic material; some have hyphae; develop from spores or fragments of hyphae
      - ✓ **Unicellular yeasts, multicellular molds, mushrooms**
    - ■ **Kingdom Plantae:** all multicellular; use photosynthesis
      - ✓ **Some algae, all mosses, ferns, conifers, flowering plants**
    - ■ **Kingdom Anamalia: multicellular,** ingest nutrients through a mouth of some kine
      - ✓ **Sponges, certain worms, insects, animals with vertebrae**
- **Classification of Viruses**
  - o **Not apart of the three domains; not composed of cells**
  - o Use anabolic machinery within living hosts cell to multiply
  - o The ecological niche of a virus is its specific host cell
  - o **Viral species** are a population of viruses with similar characteristics, occupying a particular ecological niche
  - o Viruses are **obligatory intracellular parasites**
  - o Theories of viral origin
    - ■ Arose from independently replicating strands of nucleic acids (plasmids)
    - ■ Developed from degenerative cells which could only survive from within another cell
    - ■ Coevolved with host cells

D. Methods of Classifying and Identifying Microorganisms
- Provides a list of characteristics and means of comparison to identify an organism
- Most microbes not necessarily identified by the same techniques
- Most protozoa, parasitic worms, fungi are identified microscopically
- Most prokaryotic organisms do not have distinct morphological features or variation in size and shape
- **Bergey's Manual of Determinative Bacteriology** is the standard reference used
  - o Provides identification schemes based on cell wall composition, differential staining, O_2 needs, morphology, biochemical testing, etc.
- The source and habitat of an isolate are considered part of the identification process
  - o Organism placed in **transport medium**: usually not nutritive: designed to prolong viability, used in clinical microbiology

E. Methods for Classification of Microorganisms
- **Morphological Characteristics**
  - o Anatomic details
  - o Structures (endospores, flagella)
  - o Size, intracellular structures

- **Differential Staining**
  - ○ **Gram stain: gram positive (+) or gram negative (-); Acid-fast stain (AFB)**
    - ▪ Both based on chemical composition of cell wall
- **Biochemical Tests**
  - ○ Specifically identifies **enzymatic activities**
    - ▪ **Fermenters**: ability to ferment selected carbohydrates
    - ▪ Bacteria which can **fix nitrogen gas or oxidize elemental sulfur**
    - ▪ Bacteria which produce **acid and gas**
    - ▪ Use of **selective and differential media**
  - ○ **Rapid identification methods**
    - ▪ Developed for fast identification in laboratories
    - ▪ Manufactured for **groups** of medically important bacteria
    - ▪ Perform several biochemical test simultaneously with results within 4 to 24 hours
    - ▪ Sometimes called **numerical identification**: results of each test assigned a number
    - ▪ Computerized interpretation of results is essential
- **Serology**
  - ○ The science that **studies blood serum and immune responses** evident in the serum
  - ○ Microbes are **antigenic** stimulating body to produce **antibodies**
  - ○ Solutions of such antibodies (**antiserum;** plural: **antisera)** are used in identifying microorganisms
    - ▪ **Slide agglutination test**
      - ✓ Unknown microbe placed in a drop of saline and added to several slides
      - ✓ Add different known antiserum
      - ✓ Unknown microbe will **agglutinate** (clump) when mixed with antibodies
        - ❖ **Positive agglutination test**
    - ▪ **Serological testing**
      - ✓ **Differentiates not only microbial species, but strains within species**
      - ✓ Strains with different antigens **called serotypes, serovars, or biovars**
        - ❖ Different antigens in the cell walls of various serotypes stimulate formation of different antibodies
    - ▪ **ELISA (enzyme-linked immunosorbent assay)**
      - ✓ Fast; read by a computer scanner
        - ❖ **Direct ELISA**
          *Known antibodies placed in and adhere to **wells of a microplate**; unknown bacteria added
          *Reaction between known antibody and bacterium leads to identification
          *Used in **AIDS testing** to detect presence of antibodies against HIV
    - ▪ **Western Blotting**
      - ✓ Identifies bacterial antigens in patients serum **separated by electrophoresis**
        - ❖ Proteins from known bacterium or virus separated by electric current
        - ❖ Proteins transferred to a filter
        - ❖ Patient's serum washed over filter
        - ❖ If patient has antibodies to one of the proteins, antibody and protein will combine
        - ❖ Anti-human serum linked to an enzyme washed over filter
        - ❖ This is seen as a colored band on the filter after addition of the enzyme's substrate
      - ✓ **HIV** confirmed
      - ✓ **Lymes disease (***Borrelia burgdorferi*)
    - ▪ **Bacteriophage typing**
      - ✓ Test to determine which **phages a bacterium is susceptible to**
        - ❖ Plate covered with bacterium growing on agar
        - ❖ Drop of each different bacterial phage type used

- ❖ When phage lyse bacterial cell walls, **see clearings or plaques**
  - ✓ Phages are highly specialized: infect only members of a particular species or even particular strains within a species
  - ✓ Food-Associated infections can be traced
- ■ **Fatty Acid profiles**
  - ✓ Bacteria synthesize a variety of fatty acids (FA's) which are used to identify some organisms
  - ✓ Fatty acid profiles called **FAME** (fatty acid methyl ester) are widely used
- ■ **Flow Cytometry**
  - ✓ Able to identify bacteria in a sample without culturing the bacteria
  - ✓ Use a **flow cytometer**
    - ❖ A moving fluid containing bacteria is forced through a small opening
    - ❖ Bacteria detected by size, shape, surface with the aid of a laser and computer
  - ✓ Listeria in milk
- ■ **DNA Base Composition**
  - ✓ Usually expressed as the **percent of guanine plus cytosine (G+C)**
  - ✓ Compares the **G+C** content in different species
    - ❖ **(G)** in **DNA** has a complimentary **(C)**; adenine **(A)** has a complementary thymine **(T)** in **DNA**
    - ❖ The percent of DNA bases that are **GC** pairs tells us the percent that are **AT** pairs **(GC+AT=100%)**
  - ✓ If one bacterium's DNA contains **40% GC** and another bacterium contains **60% GC**, probably not related
- ■ **DNA Fingerprinting**
  - ✓ Identifies microbes by comparison of the **numbers and sizes of DNA fragments** produced by **restriction enzymes**
  - ✓ **Restriction enzymes** cut the DNA into fragments at specific base sequence
- ■ **Nucleic Acid Amplification Tests (NAATs)**
  - ✓ Used to **increase the amount of microbial DNA** to levels which can **be tested by gel electrophoresis**
  - ✓ Use: **Polymerase Chain Reaction (PCR); reverse-transcript PCR; real-time PCR**
  - ✓ Used when a microbe cannot be cultured
    - ❖ **Whipple's disease** (*Tropheryma whipplei*)
- ■ **Nucleic Acid Hybridization**
  - ✓ **A type of bonding technique**
    - ❖ **ds** molecule of **DNA** subjected to heat; complementary strands separate
    - ❖ If the single strands cooled, they will reunite forming a **ds** molecule identical to the original **ds**
    - ❖ When applied to separated DNA strands from two different organisms, it is possible to determine the similarity between the base sequences of two organisms
  - ✓ If two species are similar or related, a major portion of their nucleic acid sequences will be similar
  - ✓ Measures the ability of DNA strands from one microbe **to hybridize** (bind through complimentary base pairing) with the DNA strands of another microbe
  - ✓ Hybridization reactions can occur between: **DNA-DNA, RNA-RNA, DNA-RNA**
- ■ **Nucleic Acid Hybridization**
  - ✓ **Southern Blotting**
    - ❖ Can be used to **locate a gene** in a cell
    - ❖ Human **DNA** digested with a restriction enzyme→producing fragments

61

- ❖ Fragments separated by **gel electrophoresis according to size** (electric current passed through gel allowing different-sized pieces of **DNA** to migrate at different rates)
- ❖ Fragments transferred onto a filter by blotting
- ❖ Fragments on filter exposed to a **labeled probe** (short segments of **ssDNA** that are complimentary to the desired gene)
- ❖ **Probe** will hybridize with a short sequence on the gene
- ❖ Fragment containing gene of interest identified by band on the filter
  - ■ **DNA Chips (or Microarray)**
    - ❖ Used to identify a gene that is unique to the pathogen
    - ❖ **Composed of DNA probes**
    - ❖ Sample containing **DNA from unknown microbe** is labeled **with a fluorescent dye** and added to the chip
    - ❖ Hybridization between **probe DNA and DNA** in sample detected by fluorescence
  - ■ **Ribotyping and Ribosomal RNA (rRNA) Sequencing**
    - ✓ Used to determine the phylogenetic relationships among organisms
    - ✓ All cells contain **ribosomes**
    - ✓ **rRNA** used most often is a part of the smaller portion of ribosomes
    - ✓ Cells do not have to be cultured in the laboratory
    - ✓ Base sequences in **rRNA** used to classify microbes
  - ■ **Fluorescent In Situ Hybridization (FISH)**
    - ✓ Fluorescent dye-labeled RNA or DNA probes **used to stain microbes in place (or in situ)**
    - ✓ Cells are treated so the probe enters the cells and reacts with target DNA in the cell

F. Putting Classification Methods Together

- ● After all test results (morphology, diff. staining, biochemical testing, nucleic acid techniques, etc.) are done one can hopefully identify and classify organisms
- ● **Two methods** of using the information are
  - o **Dichotomous keys**
    - ■ Identification based on successive questions, and each question has two possible answers
  - o **Cladograms**
    - ■ Maps which show evolutionary relationships among organisms

MICROBIOLOGY

THE PROKARYOTES: DOMAINS BACTERIA AND ARCHAEA

A. Introduction
- In Bergey's Manual, prokaryotes grouped into two domains: **Bacteria and Archaea**
  - o Based on **rRNA sequences**
  - o Identifys characteristics such as Gram stain, morphology, oxygen requirements, nutritional properties

B. Domain Bacteria
- Relatively few bacteria cause diseases in humans, animals, plants, organisms
- **The Proteobacteria**
  - o Many shapes
  - o Most of the **gram negative (-) chemoheterotrophic** bacteria
  - o **Phylogenetic relationship in these groups based on rRNA studies;** all share common **16S rRNA nucleotide sequence**
  - o Largest taxonomic group of bacteria
  - o Five groups identified by Greek letters; bases on **minor differences in their rRNA sequences**
    #### The Alphaproteobacteria
    - ■ Grow at very **low levels of nutrients**
    - ■ Capable of inducing nitrogen fixation in symbiosis with plants, and several plant and human pathogens
    - ■ Some have **prosthecae** (stalks or buds)
      - ✓ *Pelagibacter*
        - ❖ Ocean environment
        - ❖ *Pelagibacter ubigue*: named SAR 11; most abundant living organism in the oceans
      - ✓ *Azospirillum*
        - ❖ Soil bacterium, grows near roots of many plants
        - ❖ Uses nutrients from plants and in return fixes nitrogen from atmosphere
      - ✓ *Acetobacter and Gluconobacter*
        - ❖ Both aerobic
        - ❖ Convert ethanol into acetic acid (vinegar)
      - ✓ *Rickettsia*
        - ❖ Obligate **intracellular parasites**
        - ❖ **Gram negative (-)** rod shaped or coccobacilli
        - ❖ Transmitted by insects and ticks to humans
        - ❖ Enter host by inducing phagocytosis
        - ❖ Reproduce by binary fission
        - ❖ Ususally cultivated in cell culture or chick embryos
        - ❖ Causes diseases known as **SPOTTED FEVER GROUP**
          Rickettsia prowazekii: causes epidemic typhus; transmitted by lice
          Rickettsia typhi: causes endemic murine typhus; transmitted by rat fleas
          Rickettsia rickettsii: causes Rocky Mountain spotted fever; transmitted by ticks
        - ❖ Infections damages blood capillaries resulting in a **spotted rash**

- ✓ *Ehrlichia*
  - ❖ **Gram negative (-) rickettsia–like**
  - ❖ Obligate intracellular **in WBC's**
  - ❖ Transmitted by ticks
  - ❖ Causes **Ehrlichiosis** which can be fatal
- ✓ *Caulobacter and Hyphomicrobium*
  - ❖ Both produce *prosthecae*: buds for asexual reproduction
  - ❖ Both found in low nutrient aquatic environments
  - ❖ *Caulobacter*: stalks which anchor organism to surfaces
  - ❖ *Hyphomicrobium*: found in laboratory water baths
- ✓ *Rhizobium, Bradyrhizobium, and Agrobacterium*
  - ❖ *Rhizobium and Bradyrhizobium* (both known by the name of **rhizobia**): infect and invade leguminous plants; rhizobia in roots leads to formation of root nodules; resulting in a symbiotic relationship
  - ❖ *Agrobacterium*: no root nodules or nitrogen fixation
  - ❖ *Agrobacterium tumefaciens*: **plant pathogen**; disease called **crown gall**
- ✓ *Bartonella*
  - ❖ Mainly human pathogen
  - ❖ *Bartonella henselac*: **gram negative (-)** rod causing **Cat-scratch disease**
- ✓ *Brucella*
  - ❖ Nonmotile coccobacilli
  - ❖ Obligate **intracellular parasites of mammals**; survives phagocytes
  - ❖ Causes disease **Brucellosis**
- ✓ *Nitrobacter and Nitrosomonas*
  - ❖ Both **nitrifying bacteria**
  - ❖ Both chemoautotroph: use inorganic chemicals as energy sources and carbon dioxide as their only source of carbon
  - ❖ Energy sources for both are reduced nitrogenous compounds
  - ❖ Nitrate is important nitrogen form that is highly mobile in soil
  - ❖ *Nitrobacter* **species**: oxidize NH_4^+ (ammonia) to NO_2^- (nitrites)
  - ❖ *Nitrosomonas* **species**: member of betaproteobacteria: oxidize NO_2^- to NO_3^- (nitrates)
- ✓ *Wolbachia*
  - ❖ Most common bacterial genus in the world
  - ❖ Lives inside cells of their hosts **(insects)** aka **endosymbiosis**

The Betaproteobacteria

- ■ Some **overlap** between betaproteobacteria and alphaproteobacteria (Example: *Nitrosomonas*)
- ■ Use nutrient substances that diffuse away from areas of anaerobic decomposition (hydrogen gas, ammonia, methane)
  - ✓ *Thiobacillus*
    - ❖ Sulfur-oxidizing bacteria
    - ❖ Chemoautotrophic; obtaining energy by oxidizing reduced forms of sulfur
  - ✓ *Spirillum*
    - ❖ Fresh water habitat
    - ❖ **Gram negative (-)**; aerobic
    - ❖ Motile by **polar flagella**
    - ❖ *Spirillum volutans*

✓ *Sphaerotilus*
- ❖ **Sheathed** for protection and nutrient accumulation
- ❖ Polar flagella
- ❖ Fresh water and sewage
- ❖ *Sphaerotilus natans*

✓ *Burkholderia*
- ❖ Motile by **polar flagella or tuft of flagella**
- ❖ *Burkholderia cepacia*: aerobic gram negative (-) rod; can degrade more than 100 different molecules; contaminant in equipment and drugs in hospitals; problem for persons with **cystic fibrosis**
- ❖ *Burkholderia pseudomallei*: in moist soils; causes of **meliodosis**

✓ *Bordetella*
- ❖ Nonmotile
- ❖ Aerobic **gram negative (-)** coccobacilli or rod
- ❖ *Bordetella pertussi*: causes **whooping cough**

✓ *Nisseria*
- ❖ Aerobic **gram negative (-) kidney bean shaped**; diplococci
- ❖ Inhabit mucous membranes
- ❖ *Nisseria gonorrhea*: fimbria/pili; causes **gonorrhea**
- ❖ *Nisseria meningitides*: capsule; causes **meningococcal meningitis**

✓ *Zoogloea*
- ❖ Important in aerobic sewage treatment processes
- ❖ Form fluffy, slimy masses essential for operation of the systems

The Gammaproteobacteria

- ■ The **largest** subgroup of the Proteobacteria
  - ✓ *Beggiatoa*
    - ❖ *Beggiatoa alba*: grow between the interface of aerobic and anaerobic layers inaquatic sediments
    - ❖ Resembles cetain filamentous cyanobacteria, but not photosynthetic
    - ❖ Gliding motility (slime)
    - ❖ Uses hydrogen sulfide as energy source; accumulates internal sulfur granules
  - ✓ *Francisella*
    - ❖ Pleomorphic
    - ❖ Grows only on complex media enriched with blood or tissue extracts
    - ❖ *Francisella tularensis* causes disease **tularemia**
  - ✓ **Order: Pseudomonadales**
    - ❖ **Gram (-) cocci or rods**, aerobic
    - ❖ Most important genus is *Pseudomonas*
    - ❖ *Pseudomonas*
      - *Polar flagella (single or tuft)
      - *In soil and other natural environments
      - *Many species excrete water soluble pigments that diffuse into the media
      - *Many can grow at refrigerator temperatures causing food spoilage
      - *Nosomial infections
      - *Cystic fibrosis patients prone to infection
      - *Pseudomonas aeruginosa*: **blue-green pigmentation**; infects urinary tract, burns, sepsis, meningitis
      - *Pseudomonas syringae*: **plant pathogen**

- ✓ ***Azotobacter and Azomonas***
  - ❖ Both nitrogen fixing bacteria in soil
  - ❖ Ovoid and heavily capsulated
- ✓ ***Moraxella***
  - ❖ Aerobic coccobacilli
  - ❖ *Moraxella lacunata*: can cause **conjunctivitis**
- ✓ **Order: Legionellales**
  - ❖ Include ***Legionella*** and ***Coxiella***
  - ❖ *Legionella pneumophila*: colonize in warm water lines in hospitals, air conditioners, streams; survive in aquatic amoeba; causes **pneumonia**
  - ❖ *Coxiella burnetti*: requires mammalian host cell to reproduce; transmitted by aerosols or contaminated milk; causes **Q fever**
- ✓ **Order: Vibrionales**
  - ❖ Facultative anaerobic gram (-) rods
  - ❖ Many slightly curved
  - ❖ Mostly aquatic habitat
  - ❖ Members of the genus *Vibrio*: rod shaped often curved
  - ❖ *Vibrio cholerae*: causes **cholera; diffuse watery diarrhea**
  - ❖ *Vibrio parahaemolyticus*: causes **gastroenteritis;** transmitted by raw or undercooked shellfish
- ✓ **Order: Enterobacteriales**
  - ❖ Facultative anaerobes; gram negative (-) rods
  - ❖ If motile peritrichous flagella; have fimbriae; sex pili
  - ❖ Common media is **EMB and MacConkey's agar**
  - ❖ Inhabit intestines of humans and animals; commonly called enterics
  - ❖ Produce **bacteriocins:** proteins which cause lyses of closely related species of bacteria
  - ❖ ***Escherichia***
    - *Escherichia coli*
    - *One of the most common inhabitants of the human intestinal tract
    - *Important tool for biological research
    - *If present in H_2O or food, indicator of fecal contamination
    - *Not usually pathogenic
    - *Certain strains produce enterotoxins
    - *Can cause: **UTI; traveler's diarrhea; food borne disease**
  - ❖ ***Salmonella***
    - *Most members are potentially pathogenic; can contaminate food
    - *Common inhabitant of intestinal tract of animals (**poultry or cattle**)
    - *Salmonella enteric*: warm blooded animals; more than 2400 serovars
    - *Salmonella bongori*: cold blooded animals; rare in humans
    - *Salmonella typhi*: causes **Typhoid fever**
  - ❖ ***Shigella***
    - *Disease called **bacillary dysentery (or shigellosis)**
    - *Only in humans
  - ❖ ***Klebsiella***
    - *Found in soil or H_2O
    - *Many are capable of fixing nitrogen from the atmosphere (nutritional value)
    - *Klebsiella pneumoniae*: causes **pneumonia**
  - ❖ ***Serratia***

Serratia marcescens: **produces red pigment;** found in catheters, saline irrigation solutions; cause of **many UTI and RTI** in hospitals

❖ **Proteus**

*Gram negative (-) rod with **peritrichous flagella**

*Swarming type of growth on agar

*Colonies with 'concentric rings' of growth

Proteus mirabilis: associated with **UTI**

✓ **Enterobacteriales (Cont.)**

❖ **Yersinia**

*Transmitted by fleas to rats and squirrels**; respiratory droplets**

Yersinia pestis: causes **plague, the Black Death**

❖ **Erwinia**

*Primarily plant pathogen; causes **plant rot disease**

*Hydrolyzes pectin between individual plant cells

❖ **Enterobacter**

Enterobacter cloacae **and** *Enterobacter aerogenes*

*Both cause **UTI's and hospital acquired infections**

*Both found in water, soil, sewage

✓ **Order: Pasteurellales**

❖ Nonmotile

❖ Human and animal pathogens

❖ **Pasteurella**

*Pathogen of domestic animals

*Causes sepsis in cattle, fowl cholera, pneumonia

Pasteurella multicida: **transmitted to humans by dogs and cats**

❖ **Haemophilus**

*Inhabit mucous membranes of the URT, mouth, vagina, intestine

*Requires **blood** in culture medium

*Unable to synthesize parts of the cytochrome system for respiration; need:

X-factor: heme fraction of hemoglobin

V-factor: cofactor nicotinamide adenine dinucleotide (from either NAD^+ or $NADP^+$)

Haemophilus influenza: cause of **meningitis** in young children; **epiglotitis; septic arthritis in children**

Hemophilus ducreyi: cause of **chancroid**

The Deltaproteobacteria

■ Include bacteria that are predators on other bacteria

■ Bacteria in this group important contributors to the sulfur cycle

✓ **Order: Bdellovibrionales**

❖ **Bdellovibrio**

*Attacks other gram negative (-) bacteria**

*Reproduces in the periplasm, then lyses cell

✓ **Order: Desulfovibrionales**

❖ Sulfur reducing bacteria

❖ **Obligately anaerobes**

❖ Use oxidized forms of sulfur rather than oxygen as electron acceptors

❖ The product of this reaction is **hydrogen sulfide;** released in into the atmosphere and plays important role in the sulfur cycle

❖ **Desulfovibrio**

*In anaerobic sediments; **intestinal tract of humans and animals;**
*Responsible for black color of many sediments

✓ **Order: Myxococcales**

❖ **Most complex life cycle** of all bacteria

❖ Gram negative (-)

❖ *Myxococcus*

*Vegetative cells which move by gliding, leaving a "slime trail"

*_Myxococcus xanthus_ **and** _Myxococcus fulvus_: source of **nutrition is bacteria;** eventually aggregate and form stalked fruiting body, containing **myxospores** (resting cells)

The Epsilonproteobacteria

■ Slender **gram negative (-)** rods

■ Helical or vibriod

✓ **Order: Campylobacterales**

❖ *Campylobacter*
*One polar flagellum
*Microaerophilic vibrios
*_Campylobacter fetus_: causes **spontaneous abortion in domestic animals**
*_Campylobacter jejuni_: causes **food borne intestinal disease**

❖ *Helicobacter*
*Microaerophilic curved rods with multiple flagella
*_Helicobacter pylori_: causes **PUD, gastric cancer**

C. The Gram Positive (+) Bacteria

● **Divided into two groups based on their G+C (guanine + cytosine) ratio**

● The two groups placed into separate phyla

   o **Low G+C ratio (Firmicutes)**

   o **High G+C ratio (Actinobacteria)**

● **Low G+C ratio (Firmicutes)**

   o *Clostridium*

      ■ **Obligate anaerobes**

      ■ **Rod shaped**

      ■ **Endospores** which distend the cell

      ■ *Clostridium tetani*: causes **tetanus**

      ■ *Clostridium botulinum*: causes **botulism**

      ■ *Clostridium perfringens*: causes **gas gangrene, diarrhea**

      ■ *Clostridium difficile*: causes **diarrhea**; inhabitant of the intestinal tract; occurs due to antibiotic therapy leading to overgrowth

   o *Epulopiscium*

      ■ Cigar shaped

      ■ Most **closely resembles genus** *Clostridium*

      ■ Lives symbiotically in gut of surgeonfish

      ■ *Epulopiscium fishelsoni*

   o *Bacillus*

      ■ **Gram positive (+) rods; produce endospores**

      ■ Common in soil

      ■ Several species produce antibiotics

      ■ *Bacillus anthracis*: causes **anthrax**; nonmotile, facultative anaerobe; **central endospore;** disease of cattle, sheep, horses; associated with biological warfare

- ■ *Bacillus cereus*: cause of **food poisoning** (rice)
- ■ *Bacillus thuringiensis*: **insect pathogen**; used as spray on plants
- o **Staphylococcus**
  - ■ Gram positive (+) **cocci; grapelike clusters**
  - ■ Grow well in conditions of high osmotic pressure and low moisture
  - ■ *Staphylococcus aureus*: **facultative anaerobes;** produce golden-pigmented colonies; carried in nose, on skin; produces many **toxins (enterotoxins**: food poisoning; **Toxic shock syndrome toxin-1**:**TSS)**
- o **Lactobacillus**
  - ■ Industrially important **lactic acid** producing bacteria
  - ■ Most lack a cytochrome system; unable to use oxygen as an electron acceptor
  - ■ **Aerotolerant**
  - ■ *Lactobacillus acidophilus*: in humans, located in vagina, intestinal tract, oral cavity
  - ■ Used commercially to make yogurt, sauerkraut, buttermilk
  - ■ Lactic acid fermentation
- o **Streptococcus**
  - ■ **Round or spherical;** gram positive (+) **chains**
  - ■ **Pathogenic *Streptococcus*:** produce substances that contribute to their survival (extracellular substances destroying phagocytic cells; enzymes)
  - ■ **Nonpathogenic:** *Streptococcus thermophilus*: used in yogurt
  - ■ One form of classification based on their action (**hemolysis**) on **blood agar**
    - ✓ **Alpha (α) hemolytic species:** produces **greenish** (partial hemolysis) **zone** around colonies
      - ❖ *Streptococcus pneumoniae*: pneumonia
      - ❖ *Viridans streptococcus*
      - ❖ *Streptococcus sanguinis*: infective endocarditis
      - ❖ *Streptococcus mutans*: caries
    - ✓ **Beta (β) hemolytic species:** produces a **clear zone** around colonies
      - ❖ *Streptococcus pyrogenes*: also known as **beta-hemolytic Group A streptococcus (GAS);** causes Scarlet fever, pharyngitis, impetigo, rheumatic fever; avoids phagocytosis due to **M protein**
      - ❖ *Streptococcus agalactiae*: also known as **beta-hemolytic Group B streptococcus (GBS);** causes neonatal septicemia and meningitis
    - ✓ **Gamma (γ) Nonhemolytic species: no zonal** changes around colonies
- o **Enterococcus**
  - ■ Formerly called **Group D streptococcus**
  - ■ Gram positive (+) cocci in **pairs or chains;** varied hemolysis
  - ■ **Facultative anaerobic;** grow in **6.5% Nacl** and hydrolyze **esculin**
  - ■ Live well in places of high nutrients and low oxygen
  - ■ Gastrointestinal tract, vagina, oral cavity, feces
  - ■ Hospital contaminant
  - ■ Highly resistant to most antibiotics
  - ■ *Enterococcus faecalis and Enterococcus faecium*: **both** responsible for infections involving surgical wounds, indwelling catheters, UTI
- o **Listeria**
  - ■ Coccobacilli
  - ■ Produces an **exotoxin;** nonspore forming
  - ■ *Listeria monocytogenes*: food contaminant (dairy and deli products); survives (**facultative intracellular)** within phagocytic cells; grows at refrigeration temperatures; **neonatal-infant septicemia; still births**

- o *Mycoplasmas*
    - **Pleomorphic: extremely small** (easily pass through filters)
    - **Lack a cell wall**
    - **Produce filaments** that resemble fungi
    - Colonies have **"fried egg"** appearance
    - Grow extremely well by **cell culture methods**
    - *Mycoplasma pneumonia*: causes **mild pneumonia**
    - *Ureaplasma urealyticum:* urease positive; causes urethritis, prostatitis, renal stones
    - *Mycoplasma spiroplasma*: tight corkscrew shape; **affects plants**

- **High G+C ratio (Actinobacteria)**
    - o *Mycobacterium*
        - **Obligate aerobe;** non-endospore forming rods
        - **Acid Fast positive** (cell wall structurally **like gram negative (-); outermost LPL** replaced by **mycolic acids** (form waxy water-resistant layer))
        - Slow growth rate
        - *Mycobacterium tuberculosis*: **slow growing;** causes primary and reactivational **tuberculosis**
        - *Mycobacterium leprae*: grows at cooler temperature; causes **leprosy**
    - o *Mycobacteria* **Other than Tuberculosis (MOTTS)**
        - **Noncontagious;** faster growers
        - **Atypical:** found in water, soil, cigarettes; divided on basis of production of carotenoid **pigments**
        - *Mycobacterium avium intracellulare and Mycobacterium kansasii:***pulmonary** and **GI disease**
        - *Mycobacterium scrofulaceum*: causes lymphadenitis
        - *Mycobacterium marinum*: causes soft tissue infections, "fish tank granuloma"
    - o *Corynebacterium*
        - Pleomorphic; **club-shaped** gram positive (+) rods arranged in **V or L shapes**; morphology depends on age of cells
        - **Aerobic**
        - *Corynebacterium diphtheria*: causes **diphtheria**
    - o *Propionibacterium*
        - Able to form propionic acid
        - Some species important in the fermentation of swiss cheese
        - *Propionibacterium acnes*: commonly on human skin; associated with primary cause of **acne**
    - o *Gardnerella*
        - Pleomorphic **gram variable** rod
        - *Gardnerella vaginalis*: causes **vaginitis**
    - o *Frankia*
        - Causes nitrogen-fixing nodules to form in certain tree roots (alder tree)
    - o *Streptomyces*
        - Gram positive (+) filamentous bacteria that **resemble fungi**
        - The largest genus of the *Actinobacteria*; isolated from **soil**
        - **Aerobic; asexual spores**
        - Produce **geosmin** (gas gives soil a 'musty' odor)
        - Species **produce most of commercial antibiotics**
    - o *Actinomyces*
        - Gram positive (+) filamentous rods; **Acid Fast negative (-)**
        - **Facultative anaerobes** found in mouth and throat

- *Actinomyces israelii*: causes **actinomycosis** involving head, neck, lungs
  - *Norcardia*
    - Gram positive (+) filamentous rods; **partially Acid Fast positive (+)**
    - Resembles *Actinomyces*; is **aerobic**
    - Reproduce forming rudimentary filaments; fragment into rods
    - Common in soil and dust
    - *Norcardia asteroids*: causes **pulmonary infection; mycetoma**

D. The Nonproteobacteria: Gram Negative (-) Bacteria
- Not closely related to gram negative (-) proteobacteria
- Includes several **physiologically and morphological distinctive photosynthesizing bacteria**
  - **The Oxygenic Photosynthetic Bacteria**
    - Phylum: **Cyanobacteria**
    - Gram negative (-) **photoautotrophs**
    - **Blue green pigmentation**
    - Vary in shape: unicellular, colonies, filamentous forms
    - Some species with gas vacuoles (buoyancy in water)
    - Some species move by gliding
    - Produce **oxygen** from water as they carry out **photosynthesis** (similar to eukaryotic plants and algae)
    - Many capable of fixing nitrogen from atmosphere in **heterocyst** (specialized cells with nitrogen fixing capability)
  - **The Anoxygenic Photosynthetic Bacteria (Purple and Green Photosynthetic Bacteria)**
    - Gram negative (-); generally anaerobic
    - Deep sediments of lakes and ponds
    - **Green and Purple photosynthesizing bacteria are photoautotrophs**; use light energy and CO_2; do not produce oxygen
      - ✓ **Green sulfur bacteria**: can use H_2S as electron donor, instead of water; produce granules of sulfur, rather than oxygen; representative genus *Chlorobium*
      - ✓ **Green nonsulfur bacteria**: use organic compounds (acids, carbohydrates) for the photosynthetic reduction of carbon dioxide; representative genus *Chloroflexus*
      - ✓ **Purple sulfur bacteria**: can use H_2S as electron donor, instead of water; produce granules of sulfur, rather than oxygen; representative genus *Chromatium*
      - ✓ **Purple nonsulfur bacteria**: use organic compounds (acids, carbohydrates) for the photosynthetic reduction of carbon dioxide
  - **Phylum Chlamydiae**
    - **No peptidoglycan in** cell wall
    - Gram negative (-) coccoid bacteria
    - Transmitted to humans by interpersonal contact or airborne
    - Cultivated in lab animals, yolk sacs of embryonated chicken eggs
    - **Cell cycle**
      - ✓ Elementary body (**EB**): **infectious form**; attaches to host cell
      - ✓ Host phagocytizes **EB into vacuoles**
      - ✓ EB becomes a Reticulate body (**RB**): **reproductive form**
      - ✓ **RB divides producing multiple RB's**
      - ✓ **RB converts to EB**
      - ✓ EB released from host
    - *Chlamydia*
      - ✓ *Chlamydia trachomatis*: causes **blindness** in underdeveloped countries; causative agent of **nongonococcal urethritis** and **lymphogranuloma venereum**

- **Chlamydophila**
  - ✓ *Chlamydiophila psittaci*: causes **psittacosis (ornithosis)**
  - ✓ *Chlamydiophila pneumonia*: causes mild **pneumonia in young adults**
- Planctomycetes
  - Gram negative (-), budding bacteria resembling archaea (**no peptidoglycan**); some have organelles resembling eukaryotic **nucleus**
  - Aquatic bacteria producing stalk
  - *Gemma obscuriglobus*: has **double internal membrane around its DNA**
- **Phylum Bacteroidetes**
  - Anaerobic
  - *Bacteroides*: intestinal tract; some species in gingival crevice; non motile; do not produce endospores; infection from puncture wounds or surgery
  - *Prevotella*: in human mouth
  - *Cytophaga*: soil bacteria; gliding motility; degrade **cellulose and chitin**
- **Phylum Fusobacterium**
  - **Anaerobes;** pleomorphic or **spindle shaped**
  - Responsible for **dental abscess**
- **Spirochaetes**
  - **Coiled shape;** motile by **axial filaments (endoflagella);** corkscrew rotation
  - **Gram negative-like**
  - Many found in human oral cavity
  - *Treponema pallidum*: causes **syphilis**
  - *Borrelia burgdorferi*: causes **Lyme's disease** and **relapsing fever;** usually transmitted by ticks or lice
  - *Leptospira*: usually transmitted to humans by contaminated water; bacteria excreted in urine by rats, cats, dogs, swine
  - *Leptospira interrogans*: **renal infections**
- **Deinococci**
  - Resistance to extremes in the environment
  - Stain **gram positive (+) but** have a cell wall which differs slightly in chemical composition from other **gram positives (+)**
  - Contain a carotenoid pigment (**deinoxathin**) giving pink color
  - *Deinococcus radiodurans*: resistant to radiation
  - *Thermus aquatics*: heat stable; hot springs

E. Domain Archaea
- Cell walls lack peptidoglycan
- **Different rRNA sequence from Domain Bacteria or Eukaryotics**
- Pleomorphic
- Some gram positive (+); some gram negative (-)
- Can reproduce by budding, binary fission, fragmentation
- Some lack cell walls
- Aerobic to facultative anaerobic to anaerobic
- Chemoautotrophs, photoautotrophs, chemoheterotrophs
- **Can inhabit extreme heat, cold, acidity, pressure**
- Five physiological and nutritional groups
  - **Extremophiles**
    - Halophiles: thrive in high salt concentrations (25% or more)
      - ✓ **Halobacterium**
    - Thermophiles: 80 ° C or greater

- Acidophiles: grow at pH values below zero
  - ✓ *Sulfolobus*: acidic and sulfur rich hot springs
- **Nitrifying Archaea**
  - Oxidize ammonia for energy
- **Methanogens**
  - Strictly anaerobic; produce methane as an end product; **uses in sewage treatment processes**

F. Microbial Diversity

- **There is an infinite number of life forms which we still are unable to identify**
- Microbiologists have described only about 5000 bacterial species (3000 listed in *Bergey's Manual*)
- Researchers have been using polymerase chain reaction **(PCR)** to help estimate the different bacterial species

MICROBIOLOGY

THE EUKARYOTES

A. Fungi
- Study of fungi called **mycology**
- Pathogenic and beneficial
- **Aerobic or facultative anaerobic**
- **Sterols** in cell membrane
- All are **chemoheterotrophs**
- Used for food (mushrooms); help produce foods (breads); produce drugs (alcohol, penicillin)
- Acquire food by **absorption**
- **Multicellular**, exception is yeast
- Through cellular enzymes (cellulases) fungi decompose plants which cannot be digested by animals; important in recycling elements
- Nearly all plants depend on **mycorrhizae (symbiotic fungi)** which help plant roots absorb minerals and water from soil
- Most reproduce with **sexual and asexual spores**

B. Characteristics of Fungi
- **Yeast** identification involves **biochemical tests**
- Multicellular **fungi** identified: physical appearance, colony characteristics, reproductive spores
  - **Vegetative Structures**
    - Fungal colonies described as **vegetative;** composed of cells involved in catabolism and growth
  - **Molds and Fleshy Fungi**
    - **Thallus (body):** consists of long filaments called **hyphae** (singular:*hypha*) joined together
    - **Septate hyphae: most molds** the **hyphae** contain cross-walls called **septa** (singular:*septum*) which divide them into uninucleate cell-like units
    - **Coenocytic hyphae: have no septa;** continuous cells with many nuclei
    - **Hyphae** grow by elongation at the tips
      - ✓ **Vegetative hyphae:** portion which obtains nutrients
      - ✓ **Reproductive or aerial hyphae:** portion concerned with reproduction
      - ✓ **Mycelium:** hyphae grow and form a filamentous mass
  - **Yeasts**
    - **Nonfilamentous** unicellular fungi
    - Sherical or oval
    - **Budding yeasts:** form a bud on outer surface; bud elongates; **divide unevenly**; detach
    - **Pseudohyphae:** buds which **do not detach**; form **short chain of cells**
    - **Fission yeasts :** **divide evenly**; produce two new cells
    - Capable **of facultative anaerobic and aerobic growth**
    - Ferment carbohydrates and produce ethanol and CO_2
  - **Dimorphic Fungi**
    - Two forms of growth: **mold or yeast depending on temperature**
    - Mostly pathogenic species
    - **37 ° C: yeast like**

- 25° C: mold like
    - o **Life Cycle**
        - Filamentous fungi reproduce **asexually by fragmentation** of the hyphae
        - Fungi can reproduce **both sexual and asexual** by formation of **spores**
        - **Fungal spores** differ from bacterial endospores: after mold forms a spore, spore detaches from parent and germinates into a new mold
        - **Fungal spores can either be asexual or sexual**
        - **Asexual Spores**
            - ✓ Formed by the hyphae of one organism (genetically identical to the parent)
            - ✓ Undergo **mitosis then cell division; no fusion of the nuclei of cells**
            - ✓ **Two Types of Asexual Spores**
                - ❖ **Conidiospore or conidium** (plural:*conidia*)
                    *Unicellular or multicellular spore **not enclosed in a sac**
                    *Produced in a chain at the end of a **conidiophore** (*Aspergillus niger*)
                    *Conidia formed by **fragmentation of septate hyphae into single, thickened cells** called **arthroconidia** (*Coccidioides immitis*)
                    ***Blastoconidia,** another type of conidium, **buds coming off parent cell** (*Candida albicans*)
                    ***Chlamydoconidium**: thick walled spore **formed by rounding and enlargement within hyphae segment** (*Candida albicans*)
                - ❖ **Sporangiospore**
                    *Formed **within a sac (sporangium)** at the end of an aerial hyphae, called **sporangiophore** (*Rhizopus stolonifer*)
        - **Sexual Spores**
            - ✓ Result from **fusion of nuclei** from two opposite mating strains of **the same species**
            - ✓ Organism will have genetic characteristics of both parents
            - ✓ Occurs less frequently than asexual
            - ✓ Consist of three phases
                - ❖ **Plasmogamy: haploid nucleus** of donor cell (+) penetrates recipient cell (-)
                - ❖ **Karyogamy: (+) and (-) nuclei fuse** forming a **diploid nucleus**
                - ❖ **Meiosis: diploid nucleus** give rise to **haploid nuclei (sexual spores)**
    - o **Nutritional Adaptations**
        - Fungi are chemoheterotrophs that absorb nutrients
        - Grow better at **pH about 5**
        - Almost all molds are aerobic and most yeast are facultative anaerobe
        - Most fungi resistant to osmotic pressures; can grow in **high sugar and salt []'s**
        - Can grow on substances with low moisture content
        - Require less nitrogen than bacteria
        - Capable of metabolizing complex carbohydrates (ex: lignin in wood)

C. Medically Important Fungi

- ● **Zygomycota** (or **conjugation fungi**)
    - o Saprophytic molds with coenocytic hyphae
        - *Rhizopus stolonifer,* **the common black bread mold**
            - ✓ **Asexual spores** are **sporangiospores** inside the sporangium
            - ✓ **Sexual spores** are **zygospores** (large spore enclosed in a thick wall); results from fusion of the nuclei of two cells, morphologically similar to each other
- ● **Microsporidia**
    - o **Lack mitochondria; do not have microtubules; obligate intracellular parasites**
    - o Oppotunisitic organism in elderly and immunocompromised patients

- o Causes: diarrhea, keratoconjunctivitis
  - *Encephalitozoon intestinalis*
- **Ascomycota** (or **sac fungi**)
  - o Include molds with septate hyphae and some yeasts
  - o Their **asexual spores usually conidia** produced from the conidiophore
  - o An **ascospore** results from the fusion of nuclei from two cells that can be morphologically similar or different
  - o These spores produced in a sac-like structure (**ascus**)
    - *Histoplasma capsulatum*
- **Basidiomycota** (or **club fungi**)
  - o Possess septate hyphae
  - o Phylum includes fungi that produce **mushrooms**
  - o **Basidiospores** formed externally on a base pedestal (called a **basidium**)
    - *Cryptococcus neoformans*
- The fungi discussed so far are **Teleomorphs** (produce **sexual and asexual spores**)
  - o Zygomycota, Ascomycota, Basidiomycota
- Some **Ascomycetes** are called **anamorphs** (**lost their ability to reproduce sexually**)
  - o *Penicillium*

D. Fungal Diseases

- Fungal infections called **mycosis**
- **Mycoses** generally long-lasting (chronic) infections
- Mycosis classified according to mode of entry and degree of tissue involvement
  - o **Systemic mycoses**
    - Infections **deep within the body**
    - Can affect a number of tissues and organs
    - Usually caused by fungi from soil; inhalation of spores route of transmission
    - Typically begin in lungs and spreads
    - **Histoplasmosis**
    - **Coccidioidomycosis**
  - o **Subcutaneous mycoses**
    - Infections **beneath the skin**
    - Caused by saprophytic fungi (live in soil and on vegetation)
    - Infection caused by direct implantation of spores or fragments into puncture wound in skin
    - **Sporotrichosis**
  - o **Cutaneous mycoses (or Dermatomycoses)**
    - Caused by **dermatophytes**
    - Infect only **epidermis, hair, nails**
    - Secrete **keratinase** (degrades keratin)
    - Spread by infected hair, nails
  - o **Superficial mycoses**
    - Infections occurring along hair shafts and surface epidermal cells
    - Prevalent in tropical climates
  - o **Opportunistic Pathogens**
    - Usually harmless in its normal habitat
    - Pathogenic in patients debilitated, on broad-spectrum antibiotics, immune suppressed
      - ✓ *Pneumocystis*: seen in persons with compromised immune systems; life threatening in AIDS patients
      - ✓ *Stachybotrys*: grows on cellulose on dead plants; water-damaged walls of homes; can cause pulmonary hemorrhage in infants

      ✓ *Rhizopus and Mucor*: cause **mucormycosis**; patients with DM, leukemia, immunosuppressive drugs

      ✓ *Aspergillus*: causes **aspergillosis**; seen in persons with lung disease and cancer

      ✓ *Cryptococcus and Penicillium*: both cause fatal disease in AIDS patients

      ✓ *Candida albicans*: cause **candidiasis**; vulvovaginal candidiasis or thrush; occurs in newborns, AIDS patients, persons on broad spectrum antibiotics

    o Some fungi produce toxins which cause diseases

E. Economic Effects of Fungi
- **Beneficial effects**
  - o *Aspergillus niger*: produce citric acid for foods, beverages
  - o *Saccharoymces cerevisiae*: used to make bread and wine; vaccines
  - o *Trichoderma reesei*: used to make clear fruit juices
  - o *Taxomyce andreanaes*: anticancer drug Taxol
  - o *Entomophaga maimaiga*: pesticide against gypsy moth
  - o *Coniothyrium minitans*: destroys fungi that feed on soybeans and other bean crops
  - o *Paecilomyces fumosoroseus*: kills termites
  - o *Candida oleophila*: prevent undesirable growth on harvested fruits
- **Harmful effects**
  - o **Spoilage of food** (fruits, grain, vegetables) by mold very common
  - o *Cryphonetria parasitica*: **kills roots of chestnut tree** which now grows in isolated places
  - o *Ceratocystis ulmi*: **kills Dutch elm;** carried by bark beetle

F. Lichens
- Combination of a **fungus and a green alga (or cyanobacterium)**
- Exist in **a mutualistic relationship** where each benefits
- **Green alga photosynthesize** (provides carbohydrates for the lichen) while the **fungus provides a holdfast**
- If separated, lichen no longer exist
- Inhabit areas which neither fungi nor algae could survive
- Secrete organic acids, accumulate nutrients needed for plant growth
- Found on rocks, trees, concrete, rooftops
- Three morphological categories
  - o **Crustose lichens**: grow flush or encrusted onto the substratum
  - o **Foliose lichens**: leaf like
  - o **Fruticose lichens**: fingerlike projections
- The **thallus** (or body) forms when **fungal hyphae grow around algal cells** becoming **the medulla**
  - o **Fungal hyphae**: grow below lichen body forming **rhizines** and also form a **cortex** (protective coating)
- Used as dyes, antimicrobial agents
  - o Erythrolitmin: dye in litmus paper to indicate pH extracted from **lichens**
- A major food source for herbivores (caribou, reindeer)

G. Algae
- **Mostly aquatic** (some found in soil, on rocks, trees)
- **Water necessary for support, reproduction, diffusion of nutrients**
- **Characteristics of Algae**
  - o Simple **eukaryotic photoautotrophs** that lack roots, stems, leaves
  - o Location depends on: appropriate nutrients, wavelengths of light, surfaces on which to grow
  - o **Vegetative Structures**

- **Thallus:** body of multicellular algae; consists of branched **holdfasts** (anchors the alga)
- **Stipes:** stem like hollow tube
- **Blades:** leaflike structures
- **Pnematocyt:** gas-filled bladder which cause algae to float
- **Photosynthesis carried out** by cells covering the thallus
- **Algae absorb nutrients** from water over their surfaces
  - o **Life Cycle**
    - **All algae** can reproduce **asexually**
      - ✓ **Multicellular** algae with thallus and filaments can fragment; forming a new thallus or filament
      - ✓ **Unicellular** algae divide and the nucleus divide (mitosis); produces 2 complete cells
    - **Sexual reproduction** also occurs
      - ✓ Asexual reproduction can occur for many generations, and uncer certain conditions, can undergo sexual reproduction
      - ✓ Other species alternate generations (sexual to asexual)
  - o **Nutrition**
    - **Most are photosynthetic;** some chemoheterotrophs
    - Photosynthetic algae found throughout the light zone of bodies of water
    - **Chlorophyll a** (light trapping pigment)·and **other pigments** give distinctive colors of many algae
- **Selected Phyla of Algae**
  - o **Brown algae (kelp)**
    - Macroscopic: multicellular; rapid growth rate; photosynthetic pigments (chlorophyll a and c, **xanthophylls**); store **carbohydrate**
    - Cellulose and **alginic acid:** from **cell wall**
    - **Algin: extract** from cell walls; used as thickener for ice cream, hand lotion, cake decorations; rubber tires
    - *Laminaria japonica* :**induce vaginal dilation**
  - o **Red algae**
    - Multicellular: delicately branched thallus; photosynthetic pigments (chlorophyll a and d, **red pigment from phycobiliprotein**); store **glucose polymers**
    - Cell wall: cellulose
    - Agar used in **microbiological medium**
    - **Carageenan:** a gelatinous material from a species of red algae (Irish moss: used in evaporated milk, ice cream)
    - Few toxic: *Gracilaria species*
  - o **Green algae**
    - Microscopic: uni-and multicellular; contain chlorophyll a and b; store **glucose polymers**
    - Cellulose in cell wall
    - Some produce green-grass **scum in ponds**
    - Believe to have given rise to terrestrial plants
  - o **Diatoms**
    - Unicellular or filamentous algae **with complex cell walls (consist of pectin, silica)**
    - **Stores oil**
    - Photosynthetic pigments are chlorophyll a and c, **carotene, xanthophylls**
    - Produce **domoic acid (toxic in concentrated amounts);** affected person eats mussels which feed on **diatoms;** neurological disease
    - Causes **domoic acid intoxication** (in marine birds and sea lions)
  - o **Dinoflagellates**
    - Unicellular algae collectively **called plankton** (free-floating organisms)

- **Cellulose** embedded in **plasma membrane** causing rigidity
- Photosynthetic pigments are chlorophyll a and c, **carotene, xanthins**
- Storage material is **starch**
- Some produce **neurotoxins**
    - ✓ *Karenia brevis*: **algae** trapped in gills of fish release a neurotoxin
    - ✓ *Alexandrium*: produces **saxitoxins** that cause paralytic shellfish poisoning **(PSP)**; toxin eaten by mussels or clams
    - ✓ *Alexandrium* give ocean a deep red color **"Red tide"**
    - ✓ *Gambierdiscus toxicus* causes **ciguatera**
    - ✓ *Pfiesteria* an emerging disease associated with massive fish deaths
  - o **Water molds (Oomycota)**
    - **Decomposers; heterotrophs**
    - **Colorless, white** in color
    - Form "cottony masses" on dead algae and animals, usually in fresh water
    - **Asexual:** produce **spores in a sporangium** (spore sac) called **zoospores; have two flagella**
    - **Cellulose** in wall
    - *Phytophthora infestans*: infects potatoes, soybeans, cocoa
    - *Phytophthora connamoni*: infect eucalyptus trees
- **Roles of Algae in Nature**
  - o Play important role in aquatic food chain (fix carbon dioxide into organic molecules which can be consumed by **chemoheterotrophs**)
  - o **"Algae Blooms"** : periodic increases in the number of planktonic algae, due to seasonal changes in nutrients, temperature, light
    - **Red tide: blooms of dinoflagellates**
    - When algae die, the decomposition of cells associated with an "algae bloom" depletes the level of dissolved O_2
  - o Many unicellular algae are **symbionts** in animals
    - **Tridacna,** a clam, has evolved **special organs** that **host dinoflagellates**
      - ✓ The algae proliferate in theses organs when exposed to sun
      - ✓ The algae release glycerol into clams bloodstream; supplies carbohydrates to clams

H. Protozoa

- Are **unicellular, eukaryotic chemoheterotrophs**
- Inhabit water and soil
- Have a feeding and growing stage called **Trophozoite**
- Some are part of the normal microbiota of animals (*Nosema locustae*: insect pathogen)
- **Few cause human disease (Malaria)**
- **Characteristics of Protozoa**
  - o **Life Cycle**
    - Reproduce **Asexually** by fission, budding, or **schizogony**
      - ✓ **Schizogony:** multiple fission; **nucleus** undergoes multiple divisions before the cell divides; after many nuclei form, a small portion of cytoplasm surrounds each nucleus; then single cell separates into daughter cells
    - **Sexually by**
      - ✓ **Conjugation:** two cells fuse; each cell has two nuclei **(macro and micro); micronucleus (the haploid nucleus)** from each cell will migrate to the other cell; **haploid micronuclei fuse; parent cell** (each now a fertilized cell) **separates; parents cell** later divide and produce daughter cell with recombined DNA; Example: *Paramecium*
      - ✓ **Gametes:** some produce **gametocytes**, haploid sex cells; gametes fuse to form **a diploid zygote**

- o **Encystment**
  - ■ Some protozoa produce **a cyst** which is a protective capsule (survive outside host, transport)
  - ■ Some form **oocyst**: reproductive structure in which new cells are produced asexually
- o **Nutrition**
  - ■ **Most** protozoa are **aerobic heterotrophs**
  - ■ Some anaerobic (intestinal protozoa)
  - ■ All live in areas abundant in water
  - ■ Food transported across **plasma membrane** or a protective covering called **a pellicle**
  - ■ **Ciliates** take food in by waving cilia toward a mouth like opening called a **cytostome**
  - ■ **Ameobas** engulf food with the aid of pseudopods
  - ■ **Digestion, in all protozoa, takes place in vacuoles**
  - ■ **Waste** eliminated thru **plasma membrane** or **an anal pore**

I. Medically Important Protozoa

- ● Large and Diverse group
- ● **Classification** of species into phyla **based on DNA data and morphology**
- ● **Feeding Grooves**
  - o Single-celled eukaryotes with a **feeding groove in the cytoskeleton** placed in the Excavata superkingdom; most are **spindle-shaped and possess flagella**
  - o **Lack mitochondria; have a mitosome**
    - ■ *Trichomonas vaginalis*
      - ✓ Human parasite **without mitochondria**
      - ✓ Has an **undulating membrane**
      - ✓ **No cyst stage**
      - ✓ In vaginal and male urinary tract
      - ✓ Transmitted by sexual intercourse, toilet facilities, towels
      - ✓ Causes vaginitis, urethritis
    - ■ *Giardia lamblia (sometimes called G. intestinalis or G. duodenialis)*
      - ✓ Parasite **without mitochondria**
      - ✓ Have 2 nuclei and 8 flagella
      - ✓ Found in small intestine of humans and other mammals
      - ✓ Excreted in feces as **a cyst**
      - ✓ Causes fecal contamination of water
      - ✓ Causes enteritis
      - ✓ Diagnosis usually by identifying cyst in stool
  - o **Euglenozoa**
    - ■ **Euglenoids**
      - ✓ Flagellated cells
      - ✓ **Disc-shaped mitochondria**
      - ✓ **Absense of sexual reproduction**
      - ✓ **Photoautotrophs**
      - ✓ **Pellicle** (semi rigid plasma membrane)
      - ✓ **Flagellum at anterior end**
      - ✓ Most have a **"red eyespot"** (organelle which senses light and directs cell)
      - ✓ Some are facultative chemoheterotrophs
      - ✓ **Ingest thru a cytosome**
    - ■ **Hemoflagellates (blood parasites)**
      - ✓ Flagellated cells
      - ✓ **Disc-shaped mitochondria**
      - ✓ **Absence of sexual reproduction**

- ✓ Transmitted by the bites of blood-feeding insects
- ✓ Long slender bodies and an undulating membrane
- ✓ *Trypanosoma brucei*: transmitted by **the tsetse fly**; **African sleeping sickness**
- ✓ *Trypanosoma cruzi*: transmitted by the **"kissing bug"**; **Chaga's disease**

- o **Amoebae**
  - ■ Movement by **pseudopods** (projections of cytoplasm)
  - ■ *Entamoeba dispar*: **nonpathogenic and the most common**
  - ■ *Entamoeba histolytica*: **only pathogen in the human intestine**; causes **amoebic dysentery**; uses proteins called **lectins** which attach to the galactose of the plasma membrane; causes cell lysis; transmitted between humans through ingestion of **cysts excreted in feces**
  - ■ *Acanthamoeba*: infects the cornea causing blindness
  - ■ *Balamuthia* :causes abscess in brain

- o **Apicomplexa**
  - ■ **Nonmotile** in mature forms
  - ■ **Obligate intracellular parasites**
  - ■ Special organelles at tip of cell contains enzymes used to penetrate hosts tissue
  - ■ Complex life cycle involving transmission between several hosts
  - ■ *Plasmodium*: causes **malaria**
    - ✓ **Asexual phase: takes place in the liver and red blood cells of human host**
      - ❖ **Anopheles** carrying infective stage (called **sporozoite**) bites human
      - ❖ **Sporozoites** injected into human and undergoes **schizogony** in liver cell, producing **merozoites**
      - ❖ **Merozoite** infect red blood cells
      - ❖ **Merozoites** develop into **ring stage** in red blood cells (resembles a ring within the red blood on smear)
      - ❖ **Ring stage develops** and grows producing **more merozoites**
      - ❖ Red blood cells eventually rupture releasing more **merozoites**
      - ❖ Some merozoites infect new red blood cells; some **merozoites develop into male and female gametocytes**
      - ❖ **Gametes** can be picked up **by the bite of another Anopheles mosquito**
      - ❖ **Gametes then** enter into mosquito's intestine and begin **their sexual cycle**
    - ✓ **Sexual phase: takes place in the intestine of the anopheles mosquito forming a zygote**
      - ❖ Progeny can be injected into a new human host by the biting mosquito
      - ❖ **Zygote forms an oocyte**; cell division occurs; **asexual sporozoites formed**
      - ❖ Oocyte ruptures; sporozoites migrate to salivary gland of mosquito; cycle begins again
    - ✓ Defintive host: **mosquito** (houses **sexually reproducing stage**)
    - ✓ Intermediate host: **human** (undergoes **asexual reproduction**)
    - ✓ Diagnosed by blood smears
  - ■ *Babesia microti*
    - ✓ **Parasite of red blood cells**
    - ✓ Causes fever and anemia in immunosuppressive patients
    - ✓ Transmitted by tick (*Ixodes scapularis*)
  - ■ *Toxoplasma gondii*
    - ✓ Intracellular parasite of humans
    - ✓ Life cycle involves **domestic cats**
    - ✓ The trophozoites **(called tachyzoites)** reproduce **sexually and asexually** in an infected cat
    - ✓ The **oocytes,** each containing **8 sporozoites** are excreted in the feces

- ✓ If **oocyst ingested** by humans or other animals, **sporozoites emerge as trophozoites**, which can reproduce in new host
- ✓ Dangerous to pregnant women: causes congenital infections in **utero (toxoplasmosis)**
- ✓ Dx: tissue examination, ELISA, ID fluorescent antibody test
    - ■ *Cryptosporidium*
        - ✓ Common in AIDS's and immunosuppressed patients
        - ✓ Cause diarrhea, respiratory, gallbladder infections
        - ✓ Lives inside cells lining the SI of cows, rodents, dogs, cats
        - ✓ **Transmitted to humans by feces**
        - ✓ Inside host cell, **forms 4 oocytes, each containing 4 sporozoites**
        - ✓ **Oocyst ruptures, sporozoites infect new cells in host or released in feces**
        - ✓ Dx: AF or fluorescent-antibody test
- o **Ciliates**
    - ■ **Cilia** shorter than flagella arranged in precise rows on the cell
    - ■ *Balantidium coli*: causes severe dysentery
        - ✓ **Trophozoites** produce proteases that destroy host cells
        - ✓ **Cysts** excreted with feces

J. Slime Molds
- ● **Closely related to amoeba**
- ● **Two taxa: Cellular and Plasmodial**
    - o **Cellular slime mold**
        - ■ **Resembles amoebas**
        - ■ In life cycle, the ameboid cells live and grow by ingesting fungi and bacteria via phagocytosis
        - ■ When conditions unfavorable: ameboid **cells aggregate forming a single structure**; some of the cells form a stalk; others move up the stalk to form a spore cap, which differentiate into spores
        - ■ When conditions favorable, spores released and germinate to form a single amoebae
    - o **Plasmodial slime mold**
        - ■ Have a mass of **protoplasm** (called **plasmodium**) with many nuclei (multinucleated)
        - ■ Moves as a giant amoeba; movement due **to muscle-like proteins forming microtubules**
        - ■ Demonstrates **cytoplasmic streaming:** moves and changes both speed and direction
        - ■ Engulfs organic debris and bacteria
        - ■ When conditions unfavorable plasmodium separate into many groups of protoplasm; each of these groups form a stalked sporangium in which haploid spores develop; when conditions improve, spores germinate, fuse forming diploid cells, develop into multinucleated plasmodium

K. Helminths
- ● Two phyla: **Platyhelminths** (flatworms) **and Nematoda** (roundworms)
- ● Freeliving and parasitic
- ● **Characteristic of Helminths**
    - o **Multicellular eukaryotic animals with digestive, circulatory, nervous, excretory, and reproductive systems**
    - o May lack a digestive system: absorb nutrients from host's food, body, fluids, tissues
    - o Nervous system is reduced: do not need extensive nervous system
    - o Means of locomotion reduced to completely lacking; do not need to search for suitable habitat
    - o **Reproductive system: complex**

- **Life Cycle**
  - Extremely complex
  - Involves a **succession of <u>intermediate hosts</u>** for completion of **each larval (developmental) stage** of the parasite
  - A <u>definitive host</u>: for **the adult parasite**
  - **Adults may be dioecious:** female or male reproductive organs **in different individuals**
  - **Adults may be monoecious (or hermaphroditic):** one individual has **both male and female reproductive organs**
  - A few hermaphrodites fertilize themselves

L. Platyhelminths
- **Flatworms;** dorsoventrally flattened
- Classes of parasitic **flatworms include <u>Trematodes and Cestodes</u>**
  - <u>Trematodes (flukes)</u>
    - **Flat, leaf-shaped bodies**
    - Ventral and oral **suckers** to hold organism in place
    - **Cuticle** outer covering to absorbs food
    - Given common names according to **<u>tissue of the definitive host</u>** in which the adults lives **(liver fluke, blood fluke, lung fluke)**
      - ✓ *Clonorchis sinesis* (**Asian liver fluke**); seen in immigrants in the United States
      - ✓ *Paragonimus westermani* (**lung fluke**): Asia and South America
      - ✓ *Paragonimus kellicotti* (**North American lung fluke**): endemic in the United States
      - ✓ *Paragonimus species* **life cycle**:
        - ❖ **Hermaphroditic adult** release eggs into human lung; sputum containing eggs swallowed; excreted in feces of definitive host
        - ❖ **Ingested by eating infected snail: <u>intermediate host</u>**
        - ❖ **Ingested by eating infected crayfish: <u>intermediate host</u>**
        - ❖ **Human lung: <u>definitive host</u>**
      - ✓ *Schistosomia* (**blood fluke**)
        - ❖ The **cercariae** (free swimming larva stage) **not ingested, but burrow** through skin of host and enter circulatory system
        - ❖ Adult parasite found in certain pelvic and abdominal veins
        - ❖ Causes disease **schistosomiasis**
  - <u>Cestodes (tapeworms)</u>
    - **Intestinal parasites**
    - **Structure:** head (**scolex**) with suckers; hooks to the intestinal mucosa of the **<u>definitive host</u>**
    - **Lacks a digestive system; absorbs** food through their **cuticles**
    - Body made of segments called **proglottids**
    - **Proglottids** continually produces from neck region
    - Mature proglottids contain both testes and ovaries
    - **Humans as <u>definitive hosts</u>**
      - ✓ *Taenia saginata* (**beef tapeworm**)
        - ❖ Up to 6 meters long
        - ❖ Ingested by cattle
        - ❖ Larvae migrate to muscle; encyst as **cysticeri; scolex** anchors and produces proglottids
        - ❖ Dx: mature proglottids and eggs in feces
      - ✓ *Taenia solium* (**pork tapeworm**)
        - ❖ Adults living in humans produce eggs
        - ❖ Humans infected by eating uncooked pork

- **Humans as <u>intermediate hosts</u>**
  - ✓ *Echinococcus granulosus*
    - ❖ Dogs and cats are **<u>definitive host</u>**
    - ❖ Ingested by deer, sheep, humans
    - ❖ Eggs hatch in human SI; migrate to liver or lungs
    - ❖ Larvae develop into **hydatid cysts**
    - ❖ **Humans are a dead end**
    - ❖ Dx: autopsy, Xrays

M. Nematodes
- **Round worms**
- **Cylindrical;** tapered at each end
- **Have complete digestive system** (mouth, intestine, anus)
- Most are **dioecious**
- **Male smaller: 1 or 2 spicules** (used to guide sperm to female genital pore)
- In soil and water
- Infection in human divided into 2 categories: **<u>Infective Egg</u>** and **<u>Infective Larva</u>**
  - o **<u>Eggs Infective in Humans</u>**
    - *Enterobius vermicularis* **(pinworm)**
      - ✓ Spends entire life in human host
      - ✓ **Adult pinworms** found in large intestines
      - ✓ Female migrate to anus: deposit eggs on perianal skin
      - ✓ Eggs ingested by host or another person exposed to contaminated clothing, bedding
      - ✓ Dx: scotch tape method
    - *Ascaris lumbricoides*
      - ✓ **Dioecious** with sexual dimorphism
      - ✓ Adults live in SI of humans
      - ✓ Feed on semidigested food
      - ✓ Eggs excreted with feces until ingested by another host
      - ✓ Eggs hatch in SI of new host
      - ✓ Larvae burrow out of intestine and enter blood to lungs
      - ✓ Dx: eggs in feces
  - o **<u>Eggs Infective in Humans</u>**
    - *Baylisascaris procyonis*
      - ✓ Raccoon roundworm
      - ✓ Raccoon is the **<u>definitive host</u>**
      - ✓ Eggs shed with feces; ingested by **<u>intermediate host</u>**, usually a rabbit
      - ✓ Eggs hatch in intestine of rabbits and humans
      - ✓ Larvae migrate; cause **larva migrans**; results in severe neurological symptoms or death
    - *Trichuris trichiura* **(whipworm)**
      - ✓ Worms spread person to person by fecal-oral route or feces contaminated food
  - o **<u>Larvae infective in Humans</u>**
    - *Necator americanus* **and** *Ancylostoma duodenale*
      - ✓ Both **adult hookworms**
      - ✓ Both live in small intestine of humans
      - ✓ **Eggs excreted in feces; <u>Larvae hatch in soil</u>**
      - ✓ **Larvae** penetrate skin; enter blood or lymph; taken to lungs
      - ✓ Coughed up in sputum, swallowed, carried to small intestine
      - ✓ Dx: eggs in feces
    - *Trichinella spiralis*

- ✓ Causes **trichinellosis** by eating **encysted larvae** in undercooked pork, game animals, bears
- ✓ Larvae freed from cysts in digestive tract; mature into adults in SI and sexually reproduce
- ✓ Eggs develop and become larvae; larvae enter blood and lymph vessels in the intestines
- ✓ Migrate throughout body; encyst in muscles and other tissues
- ✓ Dx: larvae in muscle biopsy
  - ■ *Dirofilaria immitis*
    - ✓ Spread from host to host through bites of **Aedes mosquitoes**; **larvae** injected by mosquito travels to various organs where they mature into **adults**
    - ✓ Primarily affects cats and dogs
    - ✓ Infest human skin, conjunctiva, lungs
    - ✓ Parasitic worm called **heartworm**; can cause congestive heart failure
  - ■ *Anisakines* **(wriggly worms)**
    - ✓ Transmitted to humans by infected fish and squid
    - ✓ **Larvae** in fish's intestine mesenteries; migrate to muscle when fish die

N. Anthropods
- **Animals with segmented bodies, hard external skeletons, jointed legs**
- Few suck blood of humans and other animals and transmit microbial diseases while sucking blood
- **Anthropods** that carry pathogenic microbes called **vectors**
- Diseases caused by anthropods
  - o Scabies: caused by tiny **mite** (*Sarcoptes scabiei*)
  - o Pediculosis: caused by **lice** (*Pediculus*)
  - o Rocky Mountain spotted fever: **tick** (*Dermacentor*)
  - o Lyme disease: caused by **tick** (*Ixodes*)
  - o Malaria: *Anopheles*
- Representative classes
  - o **Arachnida (8 legs):** spiders, mites, ticks
  - o **Crustacea (4 antennae):** crabs, crayfish
  - o **Insecta (6 legs):** bees, flies, lice

MICROBIOLOGY

VIRUSES, VIROIDS, PRIONS

A. Viruses
- Filterable **obligatory intracellular parasites**
- Considered **acellular**
- **Inert outside** living host cells
- **Absolutely** require **living host cells**
- Lack: plasma membrane, ribosomes, ATP-generating metabolism
- Possess a single type of **nucleic acid: DNA or RNA**
- Once **inside**, viral nucleic acids become active resulting in **viral replication**
- Contain a **protein coat** surrounding the nucleic acid
- Can synthesize **special structures** which can transfer **viral nucleic acid** to other cells
- Viruses infecting bacteria called **bacteriophages or phage**
- **Host Range**: the spectrum of hosts the virus can infect
  - Some infect: invertebrates, vertebrates, plants, protists, fungi, bacteria
  - Most infect specific types of cells on only one host species
  - Rare cases some cross the host-range barrier (Example: **Influenza A viruses)**
  - Host range **determined by virus's requirements for its specific attachment** to host cell and the **availability of the hosts' cellular factors needed for viral replication**
  - Viruses used in **phage therapy** to treat diseases
  - Viruses may have **antitumor activity (oncolytic viruses)**
- **Viral Size**: determined with the aid of the **electron microscope**
  - Vary considerably: range from 20 to 1000 nm in length

B. Structure of the Virus
- **Virion**
  - **Complete, fully developed infectious virus particle**
  - Composed of **nucleic acid** protected by **a protein coat**
- **Nucleic Acid Core**
  - **Either DNA or RNA**
  - Can be **single stranded (ss) or double stranded (ds)**: dsDNA, ssDNA, ssRNA, or dsRNA
  - Nucleic acid can be: **linear, circular, in segments**
- **Capsid**
  - **A protein coat** protecting the **nucleic acid core**
  - **Capsid** composed of proteins subunits called **capsomeres**
  - Arrangement of **capsomeres** characteristic of a particular type of virus
- **Envelope**
  - Membrane layer consisting of lipids, proteins, carbohydrates
  - Envelops the **capsids in some viruses**
  - **If capsid not covered**, virus known as a **nonenveloped virus** or a **naked virus**
- **Spikes**
  - Carbohydrate-protein complexes projecting from the surface of the envelop, on some viruses
  - Help some viruses attach to host cells
  - Used as a means of identification

C. Shapes of Viruses
- Based on **capsid** morphology
- Structure of **capsids** revealed by **electron microscopy** and **X-ray crystallography**
  - o **Helical**
    - ■ Rod or thread shaped; flexible or rigid
    - ■ Nucleic acid located in a **hollow, cylindrical capsid** that has a helical structure
    - ■ *Rabies virus; Ebola virus*
  - o **Polyhedral**
    - ■ Many-sided viruses
    - ■ **Capsid of most in the shape of an icosahedron** (regular polyhedral with 20 triangular faces and 12 corners)
    - ■ *Adenovirus; Poliovirus*
  - o **Enveloped**
    - ■ Roughly **spherical**
    - ■ Helical or polyhedral viruses enclosed by envelopes called **enveloped helical** (*Influenza virus*) **or enveloped polyhedral** (*Herpes Simplex virus*) **viruses**
  - o **Complex**
    - ■ Have **capsids with additional structures attached** (head, pin, tail, sheath)
    - ■ *Bacteriophage, Poxvirus*

D. Taxonomy
- Classification based on **type of nucleic acid, method of replication, shape**
- **DNA sequencing** allows one to group viruses into families based on **genomics and structure**
- **Order names end in *–ales*; Family names end in *–viridae*; Genus name ends in *–virus***
  - o Family and genus names are used in the following manner: Family: Herpesviridae, genus: *Cytomegalovirus,* human herpesvirus 5
- **Species** is a group of viruses sharing the same genetic information and host range
  - o **Specific epithets not used**
  - o Designated by **descriptive** common names (human immunodeficiency virus/HIV); sometimes with subspecies (if any) designated by a number (HIV-1)

E. Isolation, Cultivation, Identification of Viruses
- Viruses need living cells to grow
- **Growing Bacteriophage**
  - o Viruses which **use bacteria as host**
  - o Can be grown in suspensions of bacteria in liquid or solid media
    - ■ **Solid media** makes possible the **plaque method** (detecting and counting viruses)
    - ■ **Plaque method** mixes bacteriophages with host bacteria and agar
    - ■ Areas of bacterial lysis produced by the virus causes produces a **plaque** (or clearing)
    - ■ Concentration of viruses given as **plague-forming units (PFU)**
- **Growing Animal Viruses**
  - o Three methods commonly used for culturing animal viruses
    - ■ **Living Animals:** mice, rabbits, guinea pigs, chimpanzees, monkeys, cats
      - ✓ Animal observed for signs of the disease or killed to examine infected tissues
    - ■ **Chick Embryonated Eggs:** virus injected near the membrane most appropriate for its growth
      - ✓ Viral growth signaled by: dead embryo, embryo cell damage, lesions on membrane
    - ■ **Cell Cultures: homogeneous collection of cells** grown in culture media
      - ✓ One sees cell deterioration called **cytopathic effect (CPE)**

✓ Viruses may be grown in primary and embryonic diploid cell lines (both grow for a short time) or continuous (maintained in vitro indefinitely) cell lines

- **Viral Identification**
  o Use the electron microscope
  o Serological methods, such as **Western blotting,** most common means of identification
    - Viruses identified by its reaction to antibodies
  o Cytopathic effects
  o Restriction fragment length polymorphisms **(RFLPs)**
  o Polymerase chain reaction **(PCR)**

F. Viral Multiplication
- **Nucleic acid in a virion contains few genes needed for synthesis of new viruses**
- Include **genes for <u>structural components</u>** (capsomeres) <u>and</u>
- **Genes for <u>synthesis of enzymes</u>** needed in the viral life cycle
  o These enzymes synthesized and functional only when virus in living host cell
  o **Viral enzymes** concerned with **processing nucleic acids**
  o Enzymes needed for protein synthesis, ribosomes, energy production supplied by host cell and used for synthesizing viral proteins
- A virus must invade a host cell and take over the cell's metabolic machinery
- Multiplication of viruses demonstrated with a **one-step growth curve**
- **Multiplication of Bacteriophages**
  o Multiply by two alternative methods: *Lytic Cycle or Lysogenic Cycle*
  o *<u>Lytic cycle:(T-even bacteriophage)</u>*: ends with lyses and death of host cell; <u>**5 Stages**</u>
    - Attachment (or absorption): virus attaches to host
    - Penetration: inject its nucleic acid into bacterium
    - Biosynthesis: **host DNA degraded by virus proteins; phage DNA directs synthesis** of viral components
    - Maturation: viral components are assembled into virions
    - Release: host cell lyses and new virions released
  o *<u>Lysogenic cycle-(Bacteriophage lambda (λ) or temperate phage)</u>*: host cell remains alive; virus capable of incorporating its DNA into host's DNA
    - Attachment (or absorption): virus attaches to host
    - Penetration: inject its nucleic acid into bacterium
    - Biosynthesis: **original linear phage DNA forms a "circle"; "circle"** recombines with the circular DNA of the bacteria; this bacteriophage DNA called a **prophage**
    - Maturation: **when host cell replicates normally, so does prophage**
    - Release: sometimes **the prophage will break from bacterial chromosome** initiating the *Lytic cycle* (leads to production of new phage and host cell lysis)
    - Three important results of *lysogeny*
      ✓ Lysogenic cells are immune to reinfection by **same phage**
      ✓ **Phage conversion**: host cell may exhibit new properties (*Corynebacterium diptheriae*)
      ✓ **Specialized transduction** is possible; the lysogenic phage packages bacterial DNA along with its own DNA in same capsid; can be transferred from one cell to another
- **Multiplication of Animal Viruses**
  o Animal viruses differ in the way they **enter the host cell**
  o Once inside, synthesis and assembly of new viral components different
  o Mechanisms of maturation, release, and effect on host cell differ in animal viruses
  o **Steps shared by both DNA and RNA containing animal viruses**
    - Attachment: attach to host cell's plasma membrane (proteins and glycoproteins)

- ■ Entry/Penetration: occurs by **receptor-mediated endocytosis** (plasma membrane forms a vesicle) or **fusion** (enveloped viruses fuses with plasma membrane; release capsid into cytoplasm)
- ■ Uncoating: viral nucleic acid separated from its protein coat by enzymes
- ■ **DNA Viral Synthesis**
  - ✓ Viral DNA released **into nucleus** of host cell
  - ✓ **Portion** of the viral DNA transcribed, producing mRNA which encodes "early" viral proteins occurs, followed by translation
    - ❖ Products of these genes consist of enzymes needed for multiplication of the viral DNA
    - ❖ Most DNA viruses carry out early transcription with the hosts' transcriptase (RNA polymerase); some viruses contain their own transcriptase
  - ✓ Sometimes, after initiation of DNA replication, transcription and translation of remaining "late" viral genes can occur; late proteins include capsids and structural proteins
  - ✓ Leads to synthesize of **capsid proteins, occurring in the cytoplasm** of host cell
  - ✓ Capsid proteins migrate into the nucleus of host cell; **maturation occurs** (viral DNA and capsid proteins assemble forming **virions**)
  - ✓ Virions released from host cell by lysis or exocytosis
- ■ **RNA Viral Synthesis**
  - ✓ Essentially same as DNA viruses
  - ✓ Several different mechanisms of mRNA formation occurs among different RNA viruses
  - ✓ **RNA viruses multiply in host cell cytoplasm**
  - ✓ Attachment; Entry/Penetration, Uncoating: same process as DNA virus
  - ✓ **RNA within the virion called a sense strand** (or + strand): acts as **mRNA**
  - ✓ **RNA** gets translated into proteins which inhibit host cell's synthesis of RNA and proteins, **and** form *RNA-dependent RNA polymerase* which catalyzes the synthesis of another strand of RNA, complementary to the original infecting strand; the new strand called **anti-sense strand** (or – strand) serves as a template to make additional **+ strands**
    - ❖ The new + **strands**: may serve as mRNA for translation of capsid proteins, become incorporated into capsid proteins to form a new virus, or serve as a template for continued RNA multiplication
  - ✓ **Four nucleic acid types of RNA viruses**
    - ❖ **ssRNA + strand**: viral RNA functions as a template for synthesis of RNA polymerase which copies – **strand** RNA to make mRNA in the cytoplasm
    - ❖ **ssRNA – strand**: viral enzyme copies viral RNA to make mRNA in the cytoplasm
    - ❖ **dsRNA**: viral enzyme copies – **strand** RNA to make mRNA in the cytoplasm
    - ❖ **reverse transcriptase RNA**: viral enzymes copy **viral RNA to make DNA** in cytoplasm; **DNA** moves to **nucleus**; integrated into host DNA (now a **provirus**)
  - ✓ Once viral RNA and viral proteins are synthesized, maturation occurs
  - ✓ Assembly of particles
  - ✓ Released from cell

G. Some DNA Viruses
- ● **Parvoviridae** (ssDNA)
  - o Disease in humans caused by
    - ■ *Parvovirus B19*: Fifth disease
- ● **Hepadnaviridae** (partially dsDNA, circular)

- o Causes serum hepatitis
- o Only genus in family causes hepatitis B (**HBV**)
- o Hypodermic needles, blood transfusions, sexual relations
- **Herpesviridae** (dsDNA, linear)
  - o Nearly 100 herpesviruses known
  - o Species of human herpesvirus (**HHV**) include:
    - *Simplexvirus*
      - ✓ **HHV-1**(HSV-1): cause cold sores on skin and mucous membranes
      - ✓ **HHV-2**(HSV-2): sexually transmitted, affects genital and lip area
    - *Varicellovirus*
      - ✓ **HHV-3**: causes chicken-pox in the acute phase; shingles in the latent phase
    - *Lymphocryptovirus*
      - ✓ **HHV-4** (Epstein-Barr Virus/EBV): causes infectious mononucleosis
    - *Cytomegalovirus*
      - ✓ **HHV-5** (CMV): causes CMV inclusion disease; seen in immunocompromised and AID
    - *Roseolovirus*
      - ✓ **HHV-6**: causes roseola
      - ✓ **HHV-7**: causes measle like rashes
    - *Rhadinovirus*
      - ✓ **HHV-8**: causes Kaposi's sarcoma
- **Papillomaviridae** (dsDNA, circular)
  - o Species include:
    - *Papillomavirus*
      - ✓ HPV: cause warts and tumors; can transform cells causing cancer
- **Poxviridae** (dsDNA, circular)
    - *Poxvirus* includes: smallpox, cowpox, molluscum contagiosum
- **Adenoviridae** (dsDNA, linear)
    - *Adenovirus*: cause upper RI, conjunctivitis, diarrhea, the common cold

H. Some RNA Viruses
- **Picornaviridae** (+ sense, ssRNA)
  - o Naked
    - *Poliovirus*: aseptic meningitis; paralytic polio
    - *ECHO virus*: fever and rash
    - *Enterovirus*: ingestion; diarrhea)
    - *Coxsackie A*: (hand, foot, mouth disease) *and Coxsackie B*:(myocarditis)
    - *Rhinovirus*: common cold
    - *Herpatovirus*: Hepatitis A virus (HAV): Hepatitis; fecal-oral route
- **Togaviridae** (+ sense, ssRNA)
  - o Enveloped
    - *Arboviruses* (EEE, WEE, VEE): encephalitis
    - *Rubella virus*: German measles
- **Rhabdoviridae** (-sense ssRNA)
  - o *Lyssavirus*
    - *Rhabdovirus*: rabies
- **Reoviridae** (dsRNA)
  - o Inhabit respiratory and enteric systems of humans
    - *Reovirus*: gastroenteritis, common cold
- **Retroviridae** (+ sense ssRNA)

- o Carry **reverse transcriptase: enzyme** which uses viral RNA as a template to make complementary dsDNA and degrades original viral RNA; viral DNA integrated into host chromosome **(provirus)**
- o *Lentivirus*
  - ■ Human Immunodeficiency Virus (HIV): attacks T-cells; opportunistic infections; often results in AIDS; Kaposi's Sarcoma
- o *Oncovirus*
  - ■ Human T-cell leukemia/lymphotrophic (HTLV): cause cancer **(oncogenic)**
- **Orthomyxovirus (- sense ssRNA)**
  - o *Influenza A, B, C*: causes influenza (flu); can lead to Reyes Syndrome or Guillain-Barre Syndrome
- **Paramyxoviridae (- stranded ssRNA)**
  - o *Parainfluenza virus*: croup in infants
  - o *Mumps virus*: mumps
  - o *Measles virus (Rubeola)*: measles; Koplik spots
  - o *Respiratory syncytial virus (RSV)*: respiratory; colds
- **Filoviridae (-ssRNA)**
  - o *Ebola virus*: fatal hemorrhagic fever

I. Viruses and Cancer
- Several cancers are known to be caused by viruses
  - o Sarcomas
  - o Adenocarcinomas
- **Transformation of Normal Cells into Tumor Cells**
  - o Almost anything can change genetic material of a cell into a cancer cell
  - o These alterations to the cellular DNA affect parts of the genome called **oncogenes**
  - o **Oncogenes** can be activated to function abnormally by mutagenic agents (chemicals, radiation, viruses)
  - o Viruses which can induce tumor formation called **oncogenic viruses (or oncoviruses)**
  - o Tumor cells go thru **transformation** (acquire features that are distinct from the uninfected cell or the infecting cell that does not cause tumors)
  - o After **transformation** by the virus, many cells produce a virus specific antigen on its surface called **Tumor-specific transplantation antigen (TSPA)** or an antigen in their nucleus (called **T antigen**)
- **DNA Oncogenic Viruses**
  - o *Adenovirus*: can be oncogenic in cells
  - o *HPV*: cervical and anal cancers
  - o *HSV-2*: cervical cancer
  - o *HHV-4(EBV)*: Burkitt's lymphoma, nasopharyngeal carcinoma, Hodgkin's lymphoma
  - o *HHV-8*: Kaposi sarcoma
  - o *Poxviridae (Molluscum contagiosum)*: wart like tumors
  - o *HBV*: hepatocellular carcinoma
- **RNA Oncogenic Viruses**
  - o Retroviridae family
    - ■ Human T-cell leukemia 1 (*HTLV-1*): cancer that affects T-cell-forming cells
    - ■ Human T-cell leukemia 2 (*HTLV-2*): atypical hairy cell leukemia
    - ■ *Feline leukemia virus (FeLV)*: leukemia in cats
  - o Viruses ability to produce tumors related to **production of reverse transcriptase**

J. Latent Viral Infections
- A virus can remain latent for long periods of time
  - *Herpesvirus 1 and 2*: cold sores; reactivated by fever, stress, sunburn; reactivated by immunosuppression **(AIDS)**
  - *HTLV-1 and HTLV- 2*: increase WBC count
  - *Vaicellovirus* (chickenpox virus): changes in immune (T-cell) response can activate causing shingles

K. Persistent Viral Infections
- Chronic infection occurring gradually over time
  - *Measlesvirus*: subacute sclerosing panencephalitis (SSPE) can occur
  - *Hepatitis B virus*: liver cancer
  - *HPV*: cervical cancer

L. Prions
- Are small ***pro*** *in*fectious particles
- A defective/abnormal prion protein **(PrP Sc)** enters the cell and changes the normal prion protein **(PrPc)** to **(PrP Sc)**
- Results in accumulation of abnormal **PrP Sc**
- Prion diseases are referred to as transmissible spongiform encephalopathies **(TSEs)**; cause progressive neurological diseases
- Diseases include:
  - *Kuru*
  - *Creutzfeldt-Jakob disease (CJD)*
  - *Gerstmann-Strausler-Sheinker syndrome*
  - *Fatal familial insomnia*
  - Nine animal diseases (Ex: mad cow disease)

M. Plant Viruses
- Morphologically similar to animal viruses
- Similar types of nucleic acid
- Some can infect and multiply in insects
- Cause diseases of economically important plants (corn, potatoes, cauliflower, beans, sugarcane)
  - **Papovaviridae**-cauliflower mosaic virus
  - **Picornaviridae**-bean mosaic virus
- Plants usually protected by an impermeable cell wall; virus enters through wounds or other plant parasites

N. Viroids
- Short pieces of **naked RNA with no protein coat** ; the RNA does not code for any proteins
- Identified to causes diseases in plants, only (potatoes, cucumber)
- Some plant viruses must enter the host by wounds or parasitic insects

MICROBIOLOGY

PRINCIPLES OF DISEASE AND EPIDEMIOLOGY

A. Pathology, Infection, and Disease
- **Pathology: the scientific study of disease; concerned with etiology and pathogenesis of the disease; concerned with the structural and functional changes brought about by the disease**
- **Infection:** the colonization by a pathogenic organism
- **Disease:** occurs when the infection results in changes from a state of normal health

B. Normal Microbiota
- Animals, including humans, normally **free of microbes in utero**
- Normal microbiota are **bacteria which establish permanent residence, but do not produce disease**
- Transient microbiota present for a period of time, then disappear
- **Newborns:** first contact is lactobacilli; become predominant in newborn's intestine
- **After birth:** *E. coli* and other bacteria from foods inhabit the large intestine
- **Human Microbiome Project**
  o Analyzes microbial communities called **microbiomes** living in and on the body
  o Used to **determine relationship** between changes in the human microbiome and human health and disease
- Factors determining the distribution and composition of normal microbiota
  o Nutrients, physical and chemical factors, defense mechanisms of host, mechanical factors
  o Age, sex, nutritional status, diet, emotional status, disability, climate, personal hygiene, lifestyle, and many other factors
- **Relationships Between Normal Microbiota and Host**
  o **Microbial antagonism (or competitive exclusion):** normal microbiota can benefit the host by preventing overgrowth of harmful microbes
    ■ When this balance is upset, disease can occur
      ✓ *Candida albicans* (vagina):
      ✓ *E. coli* (large intestine):
      ✓ *Clostridium difficile* (large intestine):
  o **Symbiosis:** the relationship between normal microbiota and the host
    ■ **Commensalism:** one benefits, the other unaffected
      ✓ *Staphylococcus epidermidis*(skin); corynebacteria (eye surface): all live on secretions and sloughed cells; no harm to host
    ■ **Mutualism:** both organisms benefit
      ✓ *E. coli* (synthesize K and some B vitamins) in large intestine; large intestine provides nutrients for *E. coli*
    ■ **Parasitism:** one organism benefits at the expense of the other
      ✓ Many disease causing microorganisms
- **Opportunistic Microorganisms**
  o Do not cause disease in their normal environment, but may cause disease in a different environment
    ■ *E. coli*: harmless in large intestine but can cause disease if it gains access to other sites (lungs, urinary tract, wounds, brain); then considered **opportunistic pathogen**

93

- ▪ *Pneumocystis jirovecii*: immune system suppressed
- ▪ *Streptococcus pneumonia*: normal residence in nose and throat; can cause pneumonia
- **Cooperation Among Microorganisms**
  - o Can cause disease
  - o One microbe can make it possible for another microorganism to cause a disease
    - ▪ Oral *Streptococci* colonizing teeth

C. The Etiology of Infectious Diseases

- **Koch's Postulates**: provides a framework for the study of the etiology of an infectious disease
  - o The same pathogen must be present in every case
  - o The pathogen must be isolated from diseased host and grown in pure culture
  - o The pathogen from the pure culture must cause same disease when inoculated into a healthy host
  - o The pathogen must be isolated from the inoculated animal and shown to be the original organism
- **Exceptions to Koch's Postulates**
  - o Some microbes have unique culture requirements
    - ▪ *Mycobacterium leprae*: never been grown on artificial media
  - o Some diseases have unique signs and symptoms
    - ▪ *Clostridium tetani*: tenanus
  - o Some diseases are caused by a variety of microbes
    - ▪ Nephritis, Pneumonia
  - o Some pathogens cause several different diseases
    - ▪ *Streptococcus pyogenes*
  - o Some pathogens cause disease in humans only
    - ▪ HIV

D. Classifying Infectious Diseases

- Diseases affecting the body lead to alterations in structure and function of the body
  - o **Symptoms**: changes in body function (pain, malaise)
  - o **Signs: objective**; fever, swelling
  - o **Syndrome**: a specific group of signs and symptoms
  - o **Communicable disease**: disease spreads from one host to another (chickenpox)
  - o **Contagious disease:** easily spread (measles)
  - o **Noncommunicable disease:** caused by microbes that normally inhabit the body and occasionally produce disease; not spread from host to another (tetanus)
- **Occurrence of a Disease**
  - o **Incidence:** the number of persons contracting the disease during a certain time; indicates the spread of the disease
    - ▪ Incidence of AIDS in the United States in 2007 was 56,300
  - o **Prevalence:** the number of cases in a population who develop the disease at a **specified time**, despite when it first appeared; takes into account old and new cases **and** how serious and how long a disease affects a population
    - ▪ The prevalence of AID in that same year was estimated to be 1,185,000
  - o **Sporadic: disease occurs occasionally**
    - ▪ Typhoid fever
  - o **Endemic: disease constantly present in a population**
    - ▪ Common cold
  - o **Epidemic: disease in which many people in a certain area acquire a certain disease in a short period**
    - ▪ Influenza
  - o **Pandemic: an epidemic disease that occurs worldwide**

- AIDS
- **Duration or Severity of a Disease**
  - o **Acute:** develops rapidly, but lasts a short time (Influenza)
  - o **Chronic:** develops slowly, disease is continual for a long period of time (Hepatitis B)
  - o **Subacute:** between acute and chronic (Sclerosing pan encephalitis)
  - o **Latent:** causative agent remains dormant or inactive for a time, then becomes active (Varicella virus)
  - o **Herd immunity:** exist when many immune people are present in a community
- **Extent of Host Involvement**
  - o A way to classify the extent at which the body **is infected**
    - **Local:** infection limited to small area of the body (abscess)
    - **Systemic (generalized):** infection spread throughout the body (measles)
    - **Focal:** local infection spread to specific parts of the body and are confined (teeth, tonsils)
    - **Bacteremia:** bacteria in the blood
    - **Sepsis:** inflammatory condition; bacteria or toxin spread and multiply in the blood
    - **Toxemia:** toxins in the blood
    - **Viremia:** viruses in the blood
    - **Primary infection:** an acute infection causing the initial illness
    - **Secondary infection:** caused by an opportunistic pathogen after the primary infection has weakened the body's defenses (*Pneumocystis pneumonia*)
    - **Subclinical infection:** does not cause noticeable illness (Hepatitis A)

E. Patterns of Disease

- A sequence of events usually occurs during infection and disease
- For infection to occur, there must be a reservoir of infection as a source of pathogens
- The pathogen must be transmitted to a susceptible host
- Pathogen must invade host and multiply
- Pathogen injures host through process called pathogenesis
- Extent of injury depends on degree host cells are damaged
- Occurrence of the disease depends on
  - o **Predisposing Factors:** what makes the body more susceptible to infection (gender, genetics, climate, nutritional status, emotional state, chemotherapy)
  - o **Development of Disease:** occurs when pathogen overcomes the host's defenses; sequence occurs
    - **Incubation period:** time interval between initial infection and first appearance of signs and symptoms
    - **Prodromal period:** short period that follows incubation period (early mild symptoms)
    - **Period of Illness:** disease is most severe (overt signs and symptoms)
    - **Period of decline:** signs and symptoms decline
    - **Period of convalescence:** host regains strength and body returns back to a prediseased state

F. The Spread of Infection

- **Reservoirs of Infection**
  - o Can be human, living, or inanimate objects; allows pathogen to survive, multiply, and be transmitted
    - **Human Reservoirs:** can be considered **carriers** if they harbor pathogens and transmit them to others (Gonorrhea)
    - **Animal Reservoirs:** can be wild or domestic animals; diseases which are transmitted to humans by animals called **zoonoses (singular: zoonosis)** (Rabies)

- Nonliving Reservoirs: soil (fungi, *Clostridium tetani*) and water (*Vibrio cholerae*)
- **Transmission of Disease**
  - By three principle routes: <u>contact, vehicles, vectors</u>
    - **Contact transmission:** spread of disease by direct, indirect, or droplet transmission
      - ✓ **Direct contact:** person to person transmission by physical contact between source and host (touching, kissing, sexual intercourse)
      - ✓ **Indirect contact:** disease transmitted from reservoir to host by a nonliving object; general term for nonliving object is a **fomite** (cup, bedding, handkerchiefs)
      - ✓ **Droplet:** microbes spread in mucus droplets that travel a short distance (coughing, sneezing, talking)
    - **Vehicle Transmission:** transmission of disease by a medium (water, food, air, blood, drugs, IV fluids)
      - ✓ **Waterborne:** by contaminated or untreated water
      - ✓ **Foodborne:** food incompletely cooked, poorly refrigerated
      - ✓ **Airborne:** droplet nuclei in dust
    - **Vectors:** animal that carry pathogens from one host to another; **arthropods** are the most important group of disease **vectors**
      - ✓ **Mechanical transmission:** <u>passive</u> transport on animals feet or other body parts (house-flies)
      - ✓ **Biological transmission:** <u>active</u> transport; anthropoid bites an infected person or animal and ingest the infected blood; reproduce in vector; pathogens transmitted to another host by vector

G. Nosocomial (Hospital-Acquired) Infections

- **Acquired during hospital stay or acquired in nursing home and any other health care facility**
  - **HAI (Health care-associated infection):** term used to include infections in day-day surgical centers, ambulatory outpatient health care clinics, nursing homes, rehabilitation facilities, in home health care environments
- Hospital-Acquired Infections result from the interaction of several factors:
  - **Microorganisms in the Hospital**
    - Hospital environment is a major habitat for pathogens
    - Most microbes causing nosocomial infections do not cause disease in healthy persons, but those individuals with weakened defenses
    - Examples: *Staphylococcus aureus, E. coli, Pseudomonas aeruginosa*
    - Most microbes become resistant to antimicrobial drugs commonly used there
  - **Compromised Host**
    - One whose resistance to infections are impaired
    - Broken skin or mucous membranes; suppressed immune system
  - **Chain of Transmission:** routes of transmission of nosocomial infections
    - **Direct contact transmission:** hospital staff to patient and from patient to patient
      - ✓ Changing a dressing; contaminating food
    - **Indirect contact transmission:** through fomites and ventilation system
      - ✓ Catheters; syringes; respiratory devices
  - **Control of Nosocomial Infections**
    - Mainly by using aseptic techniques; carefully handling of contaminated material; thorough and frequent hand washing; isolation rooms and wards; education
    - <u>**HANDWASHING IS THE SINGLE MOST IMPORTANT WAY TO PREVENT THE SPREAD OF INFECTION**</u>!

H. Emerging Infectious Diseases (EIDs)
- Ones that are new and changing, showing an increase in incidence in the recent past, or a potential to increase in the near future
- **75% of EID's are zoonotic**
- Some criteria for **identifying EID's**
    - Present with symptoms that are distinctive from all other diseases
    - Improved diagnostic tests helps identify new pathogens
- **Factors which contribute to the emergence of new infectious diseases**
    - New strains resulting from genetic recombination between organisms
    - A new serovar may result from changes in or evolving of existing microbes
    - Unwarranted use of antibiotics and pesticides encourages resistant microbes
    - Changes in weather patterns and Global warming
    - Known diseases spreading to new areas
    - Ecological changes brought about natural disasters
    - Animal control
    - Failures in public health measures
- The CDC, NIH, WHO have developed plans to address issues relating to EID's
    - Scientific journal worldwide (*Emerging Infectious Diseases*): documents the occurance, causes, and consequences of EIDs

I. Epidemiology
- Is the science which studies when and where diseases occur and how they are in populations
- **Epidemiologists:** determines the etiology of a disease; identifies other factors and patterns concerning the people infected; assemble and analyze such data such as: sex, occupation, personal habits, socioeconomic status, immunizations, etc.; ways to control disease
- Use three basic types of investigations when analyzing the occurrence of a disease
    - **Descriptive epidemiology:** data about infected people are collected and analyzed
    - **Analytical epidemiology:** a group of infected people are compared with an uninfected group
    - **Experimental epidemiology:** controlled experiments designed to test a hypothesis are performed
- Case reporting: collects data on incidence and prevalence to local, state, and national health officials
- The **Centers for Disease Control and Prevention (CDC):** a branch of the U.S. Public Health Service in Atlanta, Georgia
    - A central source of epidemiological information in the United States
    - Publishes *Morbidity and Mortality Weekly Report*
        - **Morbidity:** the incidence of specific notifiable diseases
        - **Mortality:** the # of deaths from these diseases
        - **Notifiable infectious diseases:** physicians are required by law to report
        - **Morbidity rate:** the # of people affected by a disease in a given period of time in relationship to the total population
        - **Mortality rate:** the # of deaths resulting from a disease in a population in a given time in relation to the total population

MICROBIOLOGY

MICROBIAL MECHANISMS OF PATHOGENICITY

A. Pathogenicity
- Is the ability of a microorganism to overcome the defenses of a host
  - **Virulence:** is the degree or extent of pathogenicity

B. How Microorganisms Enter a Host
- Most pathogens must gain access, adherence, penetrate and evade host defenses, and damage host tissues to cause disease
- Some microbes can cause disease without penetrating host (acne)
- Some diseases caused by accumulation of microbial waste products
- Pathogens enter the body through several routes called **portals of entry**
  - **Mucous Membranes**
    - Line the respiratory, GI, and GU tracts; conjunctiva
    - **Respiratory tract:** easiest and most frequently traveled; microbes inhaled (common cold, TB, pneumonia, measles, influenza, smallpox)
    - **GI tract:** entry by contaminated foods, water, fingers; pathogen overcomes HCl, enzymes, bile (poliomyelitis, hepatitis A, amoebic dysentery, cholera); pathogens eliminated with feces and can be transmitted to other host
    - **GU tract:** pathogens contracted sexually (HIV, genital warts, chlamydia, herpes, gonorrhea, syphilis)
  - **Skin**
    - **Largest organ of the body in terms of surface area**
    - Unbroken skin is impermeable by most pathogens
    - Access possible through hair follicles, sweat gland ducts(hookworm, fungi)
    - Conjunctiva: lines eyelid and covers white of eyeballs (conjunctivitis, trachoma)
  - **Parenteral Route**
    - Enter directly into tissues beneath the skin or mucous membranes when these barriers are injured or penetrated via injections, surgery, punctures, cuts (HIV, hepatitis, tetanus, gangrene)
- **The Preferred Portal of Entry**
  - Many pathogens have a preferred portal of entry; if entrance is through a different route, disease will not occur
  - *Streptococci* **when inhaled (preferred route) causes pneumonia; if swallowed generally do not cause disease**
- **Numbers of Invading Microbes**
  - Need large number of pathogens to cause disease
  - **Virulence**
    - Of a microbe expressed as the ID_{50}: <u>infectious dose for 50% of a sampled/inoculated</u> **population**
    - **The potency of a toxin is expressed as LD_{50}:** <u>lethal dose</u> **for 50% of the sampled/ inoculated population**
- **Adherence**
  - Some form in which the pathogen attaches to host at their portal of entry

- **Adhesins/ligands: surface molecules on pathogen that bind to complementary surface receptors** on the host cell; may be located on microbes glycocalyx, pili, fimbriae, flagella; majority are glycoproteins or lipoproteins
  - ✓ *E. coli*: **adhesins on fimbriae**
- **Receptors** on host cell mainly sugars (mannose)
  - ✓ *Streptococcus mutans*: attaches by its **glycocalyx**
- **Biofilms**: community of microbes and their extracellular products form a mass which provides attachment, and take in and share nutrients
  - ✓ *Streptococcus mutans*: dental plaque on teeth

C. How Bacterial Pathogens Penetrate Host Defenses

- **Capsules**
  - o Some bacteria make glycocalyx material which forms a capsule; **impairs phagocytes**
  - o *Streptococcus pneumonia, Haemophilus influenza, Klebsiella pneumoniae*: **virulence** due to a polysaccharide capsule
- **Cell Wall Components**
  - o Some bacteria **contain substances** which contribute to virulence
    - **M protein: heat and acid resistant;** found on cell surface and fimbriae; responsible for attachment and helps in resisting phagocytes
      - ✓ *Streptococcus pyogenes*
    - **Opa: an outer membrane protein**; aids in attachment **of host cell**
      - ✓ *Neisseria gonorrhoeae*: grows inside epithelial cells and leukocytes; use **fimbriae** and **Opa** to attach; then taken inside host cell
      - ✓ Bacteria producing **Opa** form **opaque colonies** on culture media
    - **Mycolic acid: waxy lipid** makes up cell wall; resist digestion by phagocytes; increases virulence
      - ✓ *Mycobacterium tuberculosis*
    - **Enzymes**: some bacteria aided by production of extracellular enzymes (**exoenzymes**) and related substances
      - ✓ **Coagulases**: coagulate (**clot**) the fibrinogen in blood (fibrinogen→ fibrin→ blood clot); clot may **protect bacterium from phagocytosis**
        - ❖ Members of genus *Staphylococcus*
      - ✓ **Kinases**: break down fibrin; **dissolves clots**
        - ❖ *Staphylococcus aureus*: produces **staphylokinase**
        - ❖ *Streptococcus pyogenes*: produces **fibrinolysin (streptokinase)**
      - ✓ **Hyaluronidase**: hydrolyzes **hyaluronic acid** (polysaccharide which hold together cells in connective tissue)
        - ❖ *Streptococcus* and *Clostridia*
      - ✓ **Collagenase: breaks down collagen**
        - ❖ Several species of *Clostridium*
      - ✓ **IgA proteases**: destroys **IgA antibodies**
        - ❖ *N. gonorrhoeae* **and** *N. meningitidis*
- **Antigenic Variation**
  - o Some pathogens are able to **alter their surface antigens or activate alternative genes**; the pathogen will not be destroyed or inactivated
    - *N. gonorrhoeae; Influenzavirus*
- **Penetration into the Host Cell Cytoskeleton**
  - o Some bacteria produce proteins which aid in their entrance into the host cell; mechanism provided by the host cell **cytoskeleton**

- o **Actin**: major component of the **cytoskeleton**; **actin** used by microbes to penetrate and move through and between host cells
- o **Invasins**: **surface protein** produced by bacteria; invasins **rearranges nearby actin filaments** of the cytoskeleton; causes the **actin of host cell to form a basket, and carry bacteria into the cell**
  - *Salmonella strains; E. coli*
  - *S. typhimurium*: "*membrane ruffling*"
  - *Shigella* and *Listeria*: use **actin to propel** themselves through host cell cytoplasm
- o Bacteria use **cadhesin** (protein which forms part of a transport network between host cells) to move from cell to cell

D. How Bacterial Pathogens Damage Host Cells
- If pathogen overcomes the host defenses, **damage can occur to host cell <u>four basic ways</u>**
  - o **Using the Host's Nutrients**
    - **Iron is** needed for most pathogens to grow
    - *Siderophores* are proteins which some pathogens secrete; siderophores **released into the medium**; take iron away from iron-transport proteins by binding the iron more tightly; complex taken up by bacterium
    - Some pathogens have **receptors that bind directly to iron-transport proteins and hemoglobin;** these are taken in along with the iron
  - o **Direct Damage**
    - Pathogen can cause direct damage by **using the host for nutrients** and **produce waste products**
    - Pathogen metabolize and multiply in cells; leads to rupture of host cells; pathogen spreads to other cells and tissues
  - o **Production of Toxins**
    - **Toxins: poisonous substances** produced by certain microbes; can cause serious and fatal effects
    - **Toxigenicity:** the ability to produce **toxins**
    - Serious effects: fever, cardiovascular, nervous, and gastrointestinal complications, shock
    - **Toxemia:** refers to the presence of **toxins in the blood**
    - Two general types: <u>**Exotoxins and Endotoxins**</u>
      - ✓ **Exotoxins:** proteins produced inside some bacteria; released into the surrounding medium; some are enzymes catalyzing certain biochemical reactions
        - ❖ Can be Gram positive (+) or Gram negative (-); <u>**most are Gram positive (+)**</u>
        - ❖ Soluble in body fluids
        - ❖ Work by destroying certain parts of host's cells or inhibiting certain metabolic functions
        - ❖ **Highly lethal!!** and **disease specific**
        - ❖ Need only a minute amount of toxin to cause disease; **exotoxin** produces specific signs and symptoms of the disease; **disease specific** (Ex: botulism)
        - ❖ Body produces antibodies called **antitoxins** to provide immunity
        - ❖ **Toxoids: altered/inactivated toxins**(by heat, formaldehyde, chemicals)**;** no longer able to cause disease **but** can stimulate body to produce antitoxins
          *Examples: vaccines for diphtheria, tetanus
        - ❖ **Naming of Exotoxins: by host cell attacked** (neurotoxins, cardiotoxins, hepatotoxins, leukotoxins, enterotoxins, cytotoxins); **by diseases which they are associated** (diphtheria toxin, tetanus toxin); **for bacterium which produces them** (*Clostridium botulinum, Vibrio cholerae*)
        - ❖ **Types of Exotoxins**: Three types based on structure and function

A-B Toxins (Type III): **Two parts, both polypeptides;** majority of **exotoxins**
  -**A part: active** (enzyme) component; **alters host cell function**
  -**B part: binding** component; binds to host cell receptor
  -Ex: diphtheria toxin

Membrane-Disrupting Toxins (Type II): **Lyse host cells plasma membrane**
  -**Forms protein channels** (*Staphylococcus aureus*)
  -**Disrupt the phospholipid portion** (*Clostridium perfringens*)
  -**Leukocidins:** kill **phagocytic leukocytes** (WBC's) and **macrophages;** form protein channels; most produced by *Staphylococcus* and Streptococcus
  -**Hemolysins: destroy erythrocytes; form protein channels;** *Staphylococcus* and *Streptococcus*
  -**Streptolysins:** are **hemolysins** produced by *Streptococcus*
    Streptolysin O (SLO): inactivated by oxygen
    Streptolysin ***S (SLS)***: stable in the presence of oxygen

Super antigens (Type I): Bacterial proteins which provoke very **intense immune response;** stimulate **proliferation of T cells** which **release cytokines; high levels** give rise to symptoms as **fever, nausea, vomiting, diarrhea, shock, death**
  -Staphylococcal toxins: toxic shock syndrome (TSS), food poisoning

❖ **Notable Exotoxins**
  ***Diptheria Toxin:** Corynebacterium diptheriae*; inhibits protein synthesis; A-B toxin
  ***Erythogenic Toxins:** Streptococcus pyogenes*; synthesize three cytotoxins (A, B, C); superantigens; damage the plasma membranes of capillaries→red skin rash
  ***Botulinum Toxin:** Clostridium botulinum*; associated with germination of endospores; toxin released by lyses; A-B neurotoxin; prevents transmission of impulses from nerve cell to muscle→ flaccid paralysis
  ***Tetanus Toxin:** Clostridium tetani*; known as **tetanospasmin;** A-B neurotoxin; binds to nerve cells that control contraction→spasmodic contractions, or lockjaw
  ***Vibrio Enterotoxin:** Vibrio cholerae*; produces **cholera toxin;** A-B toxin; A subunit causes cells to secrete large amounts of fluids and electrolytes; B subunit binds to epithelial cells →severe watery diarrhea
  ***Staphylococcal Enterotoxin:** Staphylococcus aureus*: produces a superantigen affecting the intestine→diarrhea and vomiting; one strain causes symptoms associated with TSS

✓ **Endotoxins:** differ from **exotoxins** in several ways
  ❖ **Part of the outer portion of Gram negative (-) cell wall**
  ❖ Outer membrane consist of: lipoproteins, phospholipids, **lipopolysaccharides (LPSs); lipid portion of LPS called lipid A (the endotoxin)**
  ❖ Released when Gram negative (-) bacteria die (cell wall undergoes lysis)
  ❖ Stimulate macrophages to release cytokines at high levels (toxic)
  ❖ Signs and symptoms: chills, fever, generalized aches, shock, miscarriage, death
  ❖ **Endotoxins** also activate blood-clotting proteins→blood clots→tissue death/DIC
  ❖ The **fever (pyrogenic response)** occurs due to production of cytokines **interleukin-1 (IL-1)** and **tumor necrosis factor alpha (TNF-α);** these **cytokines** carried to hypothalamus (temperature control center) inducing release of prostaglandins (which reset "thermostat" in hypothalamus to a higher temperature)

✓ **Endotoxins (Cont.)**
  ❖ **Shock:** refers to any life-threatening drop of blood pressure; **Septic shock:** caused by bacteria; Gram negative (-) bacteria cause **endotoxic shock**

> ❖ **Endotoxins:** cause fever (related to secretion of cytokines by macrophages): macrophages release tumor necrosis (**TNF**) sometimes called **cachectin; TNF** binds to tissues and alters their metabolism
>
> ***Capillary walls:** more permeable→ loss of fluid→ drop in blood pressure (affecting kidneys, lungs, GI tract, heart) →**shock; blood-brain barrier (CNS)** weakens→ infections
>
> ❖ **Endotoxins:** do not promote formation of effective antitoxins (due to carbohydrate component of outer membrane)
>
> ❖ **Notable Microbes producing endotoxins:** *Salmonella typhi, Proteus spp., Neisseria meningitides*
>
> ❖ Test used to identify the presence of **endotoxins: Limulus amebocyte lysate (LAL)**

- **Plasmids, Lysogeny, and Pathogenicity**
  - **Plasmids:** are small, circular DNA molecules not connected to bacterial chromosome; capable of independent replication
    - **R (resistant) factors:** plasmids responsible for some microbial resistance to antibiotics
    - **Virulence factors** encoded: neurotoxin, heat-labile enterotoxin, staphylococcus enterotoxin, dextransucrase (*Streptococcus mutans),* adhesins
  - **Lysogeny and lysogenic conversion:** occurs when some bacteriophages are able to introduce their DNA into the bacterial chromosome; remain latent, not causing lysis of the bacteria; sometimes this **prophage** will exhibit new properties; the new progeny can result in new virulent factors (toxins, capsules)→immunity (**lysogenic conversion**)
  - **Pathogenicity:** some bacteriophage genes which contribute to pathogenicity: diphtheria toxin, erythogenic toxins, staphylococcal enterotoxin and pyrogenic toxin

E. Pathogenic Properties of Viruses

- Depends on accessibility to host, evading host defenses, causing damage/death of host cell while replicating themselves
  - **Viral Mechanisms for Evading Host Defenses**
    - Infiltrate and grow inside host cells; not detected by the immune sytem
    - Viruses have attachment sites for receptors on the target cells
    - Some viruses gain access because their attachment site mimics substances useful for host cell
      - ✓ Rabies virus mimics neurotransmitter acetylcholine; AIDS virus attacks "cell-specific" components of the immune system directly
  - **Cytopathic Effects (CPE) of Viruses**
    - The **visible effects** of the viral infection
    - **Cytocidal effects:** cytopathic effects resulting in **cell death**
    - **Noncytocidal effects:** result in **cell damage,** not cell death
    - **CPE's** used to diagnose many viral infections
    - A virus can produce one or more **cytopathic effects:**
      - ✓ Macromolecular synthesis within host cell to stop
      - ✓ Cause host cell's lysosomes to release enzymes→cell death
      - ✓ **Inclusion bodies:** granules (sometimes viral parts) in cytoplasm or nucleus of some infected cells; diagnostic inclusions bodies include:
        - ❖ Rabies (Negri bodies), measles, smallpox, herpes, vaccinia, and adenoviruses
      - ✓ Fusion of adjacent infected cells form **a syncytium (multinucleate giant cell)**
      - ✓ Changes in host cell's function: can cause host cell to reduce production of immune substances (measles virus can cause reduced production of immune substance **IL-12**)
      - ✓ Chromosomal changes: can activate **oncogenes→cancer**

    ✓ Some infected cells produce **interferons:** protects neighboring cells from viral infection
    ✓ **Contact inhibition:** most normal cells stop growing in vitro when they come in contact with another cell; **viruses** can transform host cells→abnormal, spindle-shaped cells; unregulated cell growth (**do not recognize contact inhibition**)

F. Pathogenic Properties of Fungi, Protozoa, Helminths, and Algae

- **Fungi**
  o Do not have well-defined set of virulence factors
  o Some have **metabolic products toxic to human host**
  o Chronic infections (molds in home) can cause allergic (respiratory) responses
    ■ **Trichothecenes: fungal toxins;** inhibit protein synthesis in eukaryotic cells
        ✓ Produced by *Fusarium* (grow on grains-wheat, rice) and *Stachybotrys* (wall boards)
        ✓ Causes chills, n/v, headaches, visusal disturbances
    ■ **Proteases:** may modify host cell membranes to allow attachment
        ✓ *Candida albicans* and *Trichophyton*: both cause skin infections
    ■ **Capsules:** to resist phagocytosis
        ✓ *Cryptococcus neoformans*: causes a type of meningitis
    ■ **Ergot: a toxin** contained in **sclerotia (resistant portions of the mycelia);** grows on grains
        ✓ Produced by an ascomycete plant pathogen: *Claviceps purpurea*
        ✓ Causes hallucinations resembling LSD; also causes gangrene
    ■ **Aflatoxin: a toxin** having carcinogenic properties
        ✓ Produced by *Aspergillis flavus;* common on **peanuts**
    ■ **Mycotoxins: toxins** produced by mushrooms; **Phalloidin** and **Amanitin** (both **neurotoxins)**
        ✓ Produced by the **mushroom** *Amanita phalloides* (aka 'the death angel')

- **Protozoa**
  o Their presence and waste products often produce disease symptoms in host
    ■ *Plasmodium*: (causes malaria); invade host cells and reproduce within them → rupture
    ■ *Toxoplasma*: attaches to macrophage; gains entry by phagocytosis
    ■ *Giardia lamblia*: (causes giardiasis); attach to host cells via suckling disc; digest the cells and tissue fluids
    ■ *Giardia* (causes diarrhea) and *Trypanosoma* (African trypanosomiasis/sleeping sickness): both use **antigenic variation** (able to 'trick' immune response)

- **Helminths**
  o Produces disease symptoms in host; some use host for own growth or produce parasitic masses
    ■ *Wuchereria bancrofti* (round worm): causes **elephantiasis;** parasite blocks lymphatic circulation→accumulation of lymph fluid; waste products of these parasites can contribute disease

- **Algae**
  o Some species produce **neurotoxins**
    ■ *Alexandrium* (dinoflagellate) produce neurotoxin **saxitoxin;** mollusks feeding on dinoflagellate show no symptoms; **people eating mollusk** can develop **paralytic shellfish poisoning**

G. Portals of Exit

- Microbes leave the body via specific routes called **portals of exit**
- Microbes generally use same portal of entry and exit
- **Most common portals: respiratory** (coughing, sneezing) and **gastrointestinal tracts** (feces, saliva)
- **Genitourinary tract:** secretions from the penis, vagina, urine
- Other exits include: skin, arthropods, syringes

MICROBIOLOGY

INNATE IMMUNITY: NONSPECIFIC DEFENSES OF THE HOST

A. Introduction
- **Defenses that protect us against any diseases caused be microbes or environmental agents**
- Lack of immunity: **susceptibility**
- **Two lines of defense** against pathogens
  - **First line:** skin and mucous membranes
  - **Second line:** natural killer cells and phagocytes, inflammation, fever, antimicrobial substances

B. The Concept of Immunity
- Two Types of Immunity: <u>Innate and Adaptive</u>
  - <u>**Innate:**</u> defenses present at birth
    - Provide **rapid responses**; does not involve specific recognition of a microbe; does not have a memory response
    - Components **consist of First and Second Lines of Defense**
    - Responses represent **immunity's early-warning system**; prevent microbes from gaining access into the body and eliminate microbes that do gain access
  - <u>**Adaptive:**</u> **involves a specific response to a specific microbe** once it has broken the **innate defenses**
    - **Adapts to handle a specific microbe**
    - **Slower to respond; does have a memory response**
    - Involves **lymphocytes (T and B)**
- **Innate immunity**: rapid responses activated by protein receptors (**Toll-like receptors (TLR's)**on the defensive cells **(macrophages and dendritic cells)**; **TLR's** attach to components on pathogens called **pathogen-associated molecular patterns (PAMPs)**; **TLR's** induce defensive cells to release **cytokines** (proteins that regulate intensity and duration of the immune responses)

C. First Line of Defense: Skin and Mucous Membranes
- Results from both physical and chemical factors
- **Physical Factors**
  - **Skin:** human body's largest organ in terms of surface area and weight
    - Two parts: **epidermis** (keratin) and **dermis** (connective tissue)
    - Intact structure provides resistance to microbial invasion
  - **Mucous membranes:** consist of an epithelial layer and underlying CT layer; lines entire gastrointestinal, respiratory, genitourinary tracts; inhibit entrance of many microbes; epithelial cells secrete **mucus**
  - **Mucus:** in respiratory and gastrointestinal tracts, traps many microbes
  - **Lacrimal apparatus:** manufactures and drains tears; washing action keeps microbes from settling
  - **Saliva:** helps prevent colonization by microbes
  - **Cilia:** in respiratory tract, propel inhaled microbes and/or dust upward **(ciliary escalator)**
  - **Epiglottis:** covers larynx; prevents organisms from entering lower respiratory tract
  - **Earwax (cerumen):** prevents microbes from entering the ear
  - **Urine and vaginal secretions:** prevent and move microbes

o **Peristalsis, defecation, vomiting, diarrhea:** all remove microbes
- **Chemical Factors**
  o **Sebum:** produced by sebaceous (oil) glands; forms a protective film over skin; acid pH
  o **Perspiration:** produced by sweat glands; flush microbes off skin; **contain lysozymes**
  o **Earwax (cerumen):** mixture of secretions; inhibits growth of many microbes
  o **Saliva:** contains enzymes (amylase); lysozyme, urea, antibody (IgA); all inhibit some microbes
  o **Gastric juices:** mixture of HCL, enzymes, mucus; destroys most bacteria
  o **Vaginal secretions:** acid and mucus; antibacterial activity
  o **Urine:** contains lysozyme and has an acidic pH; inhibits microbial growth
- **Normal Microbiota and Innate Immunity**
  o Not usually considered part of first line of defense; can change the environment which can prevent overgrowth of pathogens
    ■ **Microbial antagonism:** prevent pathogens from colonizing by competing for nutrients, producing substances harmful to the pathogen, altering conditions that affect growth of the pathogen
      ✓ *Candida albicans*
    ■ **Commensalism:** one organism benefits while the other organism is unaffected
      ✓ *Staphylococcus aureus*
  o **Probiotics:** the study of how live microbial cultures, when applied to or ingested, exert a beneficial effect
    ■ Certain lactic acid bacteria (LAB) can alleviate diarrhea and prevent colonization of *Salmonella enteric*
    ■ LAB to prevent surgical wounds and vaginal infections

D. Second Line of Defense
- When first line of defense penetrated, second line of defense comes into play
- **Second line of defense includes: phagocytic cells; inflammation; fever; antimicrobial substances**
- **Formed Elements in Blood**
  o Blood consist of plasma and formed elements (cells and cell fragments)
  o **Formed elements** to discuss in Microbiology are **Leukocytes**
  o **Two categories of Leukocytes** based on the presence or absence of **granules** seen by light microscopy
    ■ **Granulocytes:** large granules seen under light microscopy
      ✓ **Neutrophils (polymorphonuclear leukocytes or PMN's): granules stain light lilac:** highly phagocytic and motile; active in initial stage of infection
      ✓ **Basophils: granules stain blue**-purple; release **histamine** which is important inflammation and allergic responses
      ✓ **Eosinophils: granules stain red-orange**; phagocytic against certain parasites (helminthes); produce **toxic proteins**
    ■ **Agranulocytes:** granules not visible under light microscopy
      ✓ **Monocytes:** leave circulating blood and **mature to macrophages** in body tissue
      ✓ **Dendritic cells:** long extensions; abundant in the epidermis of skin, mucous membranes, thymus, lymph nodes; **phagocytic** and **initiate adaptive immune response**
      ✓ **Lymphocytes:** consists of **natural killer (NK) cells, T cells, and B cells**
        ❖ **NK cells:** attack and kill infected/abnormal body cells; contain **perforin, granzymes**
        ❖ **T cells and B cells:** occur in lymphoid tissues of lymphatic system; usually not phagocytic; key role in **adaptive immunity**
  o During infections (mainly caused by bacteria), total number of leukocytes increases **(leukocytosis)**

o   Other infections may cause a decrease in leukocyte count: **(leukopenia)**

o   **Differential white blood cell count:** a calculation of the percentage of each kind of white cell in a sample of 100 white blood cells

E. The Lymphatic System

- Consists of lymph, lymphatic vessels, structures and organs containing lymphoid tissue, and red bone marrow
- Lymph nodes are the sites of T and B cell activation; contains macrophages and dendritic cells
- Lymphoid tissues and organs: scattered throughout the respiratory, gastrointestinal, urinary and reproductive tracts; protect against microbes that are ingested or inhaled
- Spleen: contains lymphocytes and macrophages; monitors blood for microbes
- Thymus: site for T cell maturation; contains macrophages and dendritic cells

F. Phagocytes

- **Phagocytosis**
  - o   The **ingestion of microbes or other foreign substances** by a phagocytic (WBC or derivatives of WBC's) cell
  - o   Involves clearing away debris
- **Actions of Phagocytic Cells**
  - o   When **infection** occurs, granulocytes (**primarily neutrophils**) **and monocytes migrate** to infected site
  - o   **Monocytes develop into macrophages** during this migration; migrate into tissues
  - o   **Fixed macrophages (or histiocytes)** are resident in certain tissues and organs
  - o   **Free (wandering) macrophages:** are motile and roam the tissues and gather at infection site
  - o   **Mononuclear phagocytic (reticuloendothelial) system:** the various macrophages of the body
- **The Mechanisms of Phagocytosis**
  - o   **Chemotaxis: chemical attraction** of phagocyte to microbe; chemotactic chemicals include: microbial products, components of WBC's, damaged tissue cells, cytokines, peptides (from complement)
  - o   **Adherence:** phagocyte's plasma membrane **adheres/attaches to surface** of the microorganism or foreign material; binding of PAMPs to TLRs initiates phagocytosis and causes the phagocyte to release cytokines that recruit more phagocytes
    - ■   Microbes more readily phagocytized if coated with a certain serum protein which **promotes attachment;** coating process called **opsonization**
  - o   **Ingestion:** plasma membrane of the phagocyte produces **pseudopods that engulf the microbe;** surround the microbe in a sac called a **phagosome** (phagocytic vesicle) which pumps protons inside
  - o   **Digestion: phagosome** pinches off from plasma membrane and enters cytoplasm; fuses with lysosomes (contain **lysozymes and other digestive enzymes)** to form **a phagolysosome**
    - ■   Contents inside phagolysosome digested
    - ■   **Phagolysosome** now contain **indigestible material;** called a **residual body**
  - o   **Exocytosis: residual body** discharges/extrudes its waste outside the cell
- **Microbial Evasion of Phagocytosis**
  - o   Some bacteria have structures that inhibit adherence (**M proteins, capsules**)
    - ■   *Streptococcus pyogenes* (**M protein**) and *Streptococcus pneumonia* (**capsule**)
  - o   Some microbes can be ingested, but not killed
    - ■   *Staphylococcus:* produce **leucocidins** (causes phagocytic cells to release their own lysosomal enzymes)
  - o   Secrete **pore forming toxins** which lyse phagocyte cell membrane

- *Trypanosoma cruzi* and *Listeria monocytogenes*: both produce **membrane attack complexes (MAC)** that lyse phagolysosomes
  - o Some microbes can **survive inside phagocytes**
    - *Rickettsia*: escape from a phagosome before it fuses with lysosome
  - o Some microbes can become dormant within phagocyte for months or years
    - *Francisella tularensis*: causes Tularemia
  - o Some can produce **biofilms**
    - *Pseudomonas aeruginosa*

G. Inflammation
- A defensive response triggered by the body when damaged
- The damage can be caused by: microbial infections, physical agents, chemical agents
- Characterized by **four main signs and symptoms: redness, pain, heat, swelling**
  - o **Loss of function:** considered a **fifth** sign and symptom depending on the site and extend of damage
- Acute inflammation: if cause of inflammation removed in a short period of time, and the inflammatory response is intense
  - o Ex: boil caused by *Staphylococcus aureus*
- Chronic inflammation: if cause of inflammation is difficult or impossible to remove, longer lasting, and less intense
  - o Ex: granulomas in lung caused by *Mycobacteria tuberculosis*
- Inflammation has the following functions: to destroy the injurious agent; limit the effects of the injurious agent; repair or replace damaged tissue
- During early stages of inflammation: microbial structures (LPS, flagellin, bacterial DNA) stimulate macrophages to produce cytokines (TNF-α); in response, liver synthesizes proteins called **acute-phase** proteins (C-reactive protein, mannose-binding lectin, fibrinogen, and kinins) which induce both local and systemic responses
- Inflammatory process divided into **three phases**
  - o **Vasodilation and Increased Permeability of Blood Vessels**
    - Blood vessels dilate following tissue damage and their permeability increases; fluid moves from blood into tissue space causing **edema**
    - Chemicals (histamine, prostaglandins, leukotrienes, kinins) and clotting elements from damaged cells released
    - Can lead to pus (dead cells, fluid) formation and/or abscess (cavity)
  - o **Phagocyte Migration and Phagocytosis**
    - Neutrophils and monocytes **stick (marginate)** to inner surface of blood vessels
    - These phagocytic cells squeeze between the endothelial cell and migrate in **an amoeboid movement (diapedesis)** to damaged area, destroying invading microbes
    - Granulocytes predominate in early stages of infection; macrophages enter during later stage
    - Granulocytes or macrophages engulf the microorganisms and damaged tissue; they eventually die; pus forms
  - o **Tissue Repair**
    - Certain tissues replace dead or damaged cells
    - Repair (depending on tissue type) **begins during active phase of inflammation**; cannot be completed until all harmful substances have been removed or neutralized
    - Repair: the **stroma (supporting CT) or parenchyma (functioning part) produces new cells**
    - Fibroblasts induced by cytokines (released by activated macrophages) to synthesize collagen fibers; fibers aggregate to make scar tissue, process called **fibrosis**

H. Fever
- **An abnormally high body temperature in response to injury (infection)**
- Caused by certain substances which affect the hypothalamus (body's thermostat normally at 37^0C /98.6^{0}F)
- Endotoxins released causing phagocytes to release IL-1, along with TNF-α; these cytokines cause hypothalamus to release prostaglandins that reset the hypothalamic thermostat at a higher temperature→ fever
- The body responds to the new temperature adjustment by constricting blood vessels, increasing rate of metabolism and **shivering**
- A **"chill"** indicates rising body temperature; **crisis (sweating)** indicates body temperature lowering
- Complications of fever are: tachycardia, increased metabolic rate, dehydration, seizures, death

I. Antimicrobial Substances
- Produced by the body in addition to the chemical factors
- Complement System: important proteins are interferons, iron-binding proteins, antimicrobial peptides
- **The Complement System**
  - Consists of **proteins produced by the liver**, circulating in blood serum and tissues
  - "Complements" cells of the immune system in destroying microbes by: cytolysis, inflammation, phagocytosis; also prevents excessive tissue damage
  - Designated by uppercase C; are inactive until split into fragments (products)
  - Activated proteins indicated by lowercase letters a and b
  - Acts in a cascade (one reaction triggers another, which triggers another, etc....)
  - Activation of **C3 starts** a cascade resulting in cytolysis, inflammation, and phagocytosis
    - Inactive **C3** splits into C3a and C3b
    - C3b binds to microbe; receptors on phagocytes attach to C3b; **C3b** enhances **opsonization**
    - C3b splits C5 into C5a and C5b
    - Fragments C5b, C6, C7, and C8 bind together sequentially, attaching to microbes plasma membrane
    - C5b through C8: act as a receptor which attracts a C9 fragment
    - Additional C9 fragments added to form a transmembrane channel
    - C5b through C8 and multiple C9 fragments form a **membrane attack complex (MAC)** which inserts holes through the membrane→ **cytolysis**
    - C3a and C5a: bind to mast cells→ release of histamine→increase blood vessel permeability
    - C5a also a powerful chemotactic factor attracting phagocytes to site of an infection
    - **MAC** forms the basis for the complement fixation test used to diagnose some diseases
  - This cascade of complement proteins, **called complement activation,** may occur in **three pathways**
    - **Classic pathway:** initiated by an **antigen-antibody reaction**; antibodies attach to antigens forming antibody-antigen complexes; this complex binds and activates C1; activated C1→activates C2 and C4 (producing C2a and C2b and C4a and C4b); C2a and C4b combine and activates C3, splitting it into C3a and C3b
    - **Alternative pathway: does not involve antibodies**; initiated by contact between certain complement proteins and a pathogen; C3 binds with factors (B, D, P) on microbes surface→C3 split into C3a and C3b
    - **Lectin pathway:** ingestion of bacteria, viruses, and other foreign matter cause macrophages to release cytokines; cytokines stimulate liver to produce **lectins** (proteins which bind to carbohydrates); mannose-binding lectin **(MBL)** binds to mannose on surface of microbe→ enhancing phagocytosis and activates C2 and C4; C2a and C4b activates C3
  - **Regulation of Complement:** various regulatory proteins in host's blood and on certain cells
    - The proteins breakdown activated complement and function as inhibitors
  - **Complement and Disease:** Inherited diseases

- C1, C2, or C4: cause collagen vascular disorders→hypersensitivity
- C3: increased susceptibility to recurrent infections with pyogenic microbes
- C5 through C9: increased susceptibility to *Neisseria meningitides and Neisseria gonorrhoeae*
- Diseases such as: asthma, SLE, forms of arthritis, multiple sclerosis, IBD, Alzheimer's
  - o **Evading the Complement System**
    - Some bacteria have capsules; some surface lipid-carbohydrate complexes; enzymes to destroy C5a
- **Interferons (IFNs)**
  - o Are **antiviral proteins** which interfere with viral multiplication, produced by animal cells (lymphocytes, macrophages); stable at low pH and fairly heat resistant
  - o Are host-cell-specific, not virus-specific
  - o In humans, **interferons** produced by fibroblasts, lymphocytes, and other leukocytes
  - o **Three types** of human interferons; each type having a different effect on the body
    - **Alpha interferon (α-IFN)**: produced by virus infected host cells; diffuse to uninfected neighboring cells; uninfected cell synthesizes **antiviral proteins (AVPs); AVPs** are enzymes that disrupt viral replication at different stages
    - **Beta interferon (β-IFN)**: same as α-IFN
    - **Gamma interferon (γ-IFN)**: produced by lymphocytes; induces neutrophils and macrophages to kill bacteria
    - **α-IFN and β-IFN**: both host-cell-specific, not virus-specific
  - o Effective for short period of time; not stable for long periods of time
  - o Potential as anticancer agents
    - **α-IFN**: for Kaposi's sarcoma, genital herpes
    - **β-IFN**: multiple sclerosis (MS)
  - o Interferons produced with recombinant DNA techniques called **recombinant interferons (rIFNs)**
  - o Side effects: nausea, vomiting, weight loss, fever; some viruses are resistant (inhibit **AVPs**)
- **Iron-Binding Proteins**
  - o Most iron in body bound to molecules
  - o These molecules: **transferrin** (blood, tissue fluids)**, lactoferrin** (milk, saliva, mucus)**, ferritin** (liver, spleen, red bone marrow)**, hemoglobin** (within red blood cells) called **iron binding proteins**
  - o **Siderophores**: protein secreted by many pathogenic bacteria to take away iron from iron-binding proteins
  - o Some pathogens produce receptors on its surface to bind directly to iron-binding protein; the iron-binding protein is taken into bacteria (*Neisseria meningitidis*)
  - o *Streptococcus pyogenes*: release the protein hemolysin→lyse red blood cells; hemoglobin degraded to capture iron
- **Antimicrobial Peptides (AMPs)**
  - o Short peptides consisting of 12 to 50 amino acids; found in plants and animals
  - o Have a broad spectrum of antimicrobial activities against: bacteria, fungi, viruses, eukaryotic parasites
  - o **Modes of action:** inhibit cell wall synthesis; form pores in the plasma membrane→lysis; destroying DNA and RNA
  - o **AMPs produced by humans:** dermcidin (produced by sweat glands), defensins, and cathelicidins (produced by neutrophils, macrophages, epithelium), and thrombocidin (produced by platelets)
  - o Synergic with other antimicrobial agents; stable over a wide range of pH
  - o Can sequester the LPS shed from gram negative(-) bacteria
  - o Attract dendritic cells and initiate an adaptive response
  - o Recruit mast cells

MICROBIOLOGY

ADAPTIVE IMMUNITY: SPECIFIC DEFENSES OF THE HOST

A. The Adaptive Immune System
- Immunity means **"to exempt"**
- **Adaptive immunity:** the ability of the body to adapt to a specific microbial invader or a foreign substance; a memory of the infection
- **More specialized, genetically predetermined type of immunity developed during individual's lifetime**
- Involves the production of proteins called **antibodies and specialized lymphocytes** against a foreign substance (antigen)
- **Vaccinations:** exposing an individual to harmless versions of a pathogen that cause certain diseases, rendering the individual to develop immunity

B. Dual Nature of the Adaptive Immune System
- Consist of a **Humoral and Cellular component**
- <u>**Humoral Immunity**</u>
  - o **Production of antibodies** that act against foreign substances or organisms; defends primarily against bacteria, bacterial toxins, viruses
  - o Red **bone marrow stem cells** produce **lymphocytes**; lymphocytes that mature in bone marrow **become B cells (B lymphocytes)**
  - o **B cells** recognize antigens and make specific antibodies
- <u>**Cellular Immunity**</u>
  - o Other **lymphocytes** mature under the influence of the **thymus**; **T cells,** like B cells, respond to antigens by means of **T-cell receptors (TCRs)** on their surface; contact with an antigen which is complementary to the **TCR**, can cause certain types of **T cells** to proliferate and secrete **cytokines**
  - o Involves specialized **T cells (T lymphocytes);** regulate the activation of macrophages; effective against bacteria and viruses within phagocytic or infected cells, fungi, helminthes; transplanted tissue (skin grafts, transplants)

C. Types of Adaptive Immunity
- Adaptive immunity refers to the protection one develops against certain microbes or foreign substances
- Immunity can be acquired either: **actively or passively**
- Both **active and passive immunities can be obtained naturally or artificially**
  - o <u>**Naturally Acquired Immunity**</u>
    - ■ **Active:** obtained when <u>**exposed to antigens**</u> which enter the body; the immune system responds (making antibodies), person recovers; immunity is lifelong (measles, chickenpox)
    - ■ **Passive:** natural <u>**transfer of antibodies**</u> from mother to infant **(transplacental transfer);** maternal antibodies essential until infant's immune system matures (<u>colostrum</u>)
  - o <u>**Artificially Acquired Immunity**</u>
    - ■ **Active:** <u>**prepared antigens**</u> (vaccines) → body→antibodies and specialized lymphocytes **(immunization)**

- Passive: <u>preformed antibodies</u> injected into body; from animal or person already immune to the disease; found in their **serum (aka antiserum)**

- Terms
  - **Antiserum: blood serum** containing considerable concentration of **antibodies**
  - **Serology:** study of reactions between antibodies and antigens
  - **Gamma globulin:** fraction of globulin proteins containing most of the antibodies on **electrophoresis**

D. Antigens and Antibodies
- **The Nature of Antigens**
  - **Antigens (aka immunogens):** a foreign substance causing the body to produce specific antibodies
  - Most are either proteins or polysaccharides
  - Antigenic compounds: capsules, cell walls, flagella, fimbriae, toxins; coats of viruses; pollen, egg, blood cell surfaces; transplanted tissues and organs
  - Antibodies are produced against specific regions on the **surface of the antigen called antigenic determinants (or epitopes)**
  - Most antigens have a molecular weight of 10,000 or higher
  - **Hapten:** low molecular weight substance that does not cause the formation of antibodies by itself, but does so when combined with a carrier molecule (example: penicillin)

- **The Nature of Antibodies**
  - Antibodies are **globular proteins** produced by **B cells** in the presence of an antigen; relatively soluble
  - Use the term **immunoglobulins (Ig)** for antibodies
  - An antibody has at least two identical binding sites that bind to epitopes; sites called **antigen-binding sites**
  - The number of antigen-binding sites on the antibody called **valence;** most human antibodies have two binding sites (**bivalent**)
  - **Antibody Structure**
    - Simplest structure of a bivalent antibody called a **monomer;** consists of four protein chains
      - ✓ Two identical **light (L) chains** and two identical **heavy (H) chains; L and H** refer to molecular weights
    - Chains joined by disulfide links and other bonds to form a **'Y-shaped' molecule,** which is flexible and can form a **T-shape**
    - Two regions of the protein chain: **variable (V) region** and **constant (C) region**
      - ✓ **V region: arms** of the antibody monomer; binds to the **epitopes** (sites where antibody binds with antigen)
      - ✓ **C region: stem** of the antibody monomer; **5 major types of C regions;** stem called the Fc region; if left exposed after both antigen-binding sites attach to an antigen, Fc regions of adjacent antibodies can bind complement
  - **Immunoglobulin Classes**
    - Monomers are the simplest and most abundant immunoglobulins
    - **Five classes;** each with a different role in the immune response
      - ✓ <u>Ig</u>**G:** monomer; accounts for about **80% of all antibodies in the serum;** crosses **placenta** (passive immunity to fetus); neutralizes bacterial toxins; protects against circulating bacteria and viruses
      - ✓ <u>Ig</u>**M: pentamer** structure of 5 monomers bonded together by **J (joining) chain; first to respond to an antigen or initial infection;** large; predominant antibody involved in the response to ABO blood group antigens; involved in agglutination and complement fixation

- ✓ **IgA**: serum **IgA** antibodies are monomers; **secretory IgA** antibodies are dimers; most **abundant in body secretions** (mucus, saliva, tears, breast milk and mucous membranes); protects infants from GI infections; prevents attachments of pathogens to mucosal surface
- ✓ **IgD**: found in blood, lymph fluid, surface of B cells; **function not well defined**
- ✓ **IgE**: binds to **basophils and mast cells→histamine→**allergic reaction (hay fever); attracts complement and phagocytic cells; provides protection against **parasitic worms**

E. B cells and Humoral Immunity
- ● Humoral response is carried out by antibodies which are produced by **activated B cells**
- ● Process leading to production of antibodies starts when B cells exposed to **free, or extracellular, antigens**
- ● **Clonal Selection of Antibody-Producing Cells**
  - o Each B cell carries immunoglobulins on its surface
  - o Majority of B cell's surface immunoglobulins are IgM and IgD
  - o When B cell's immunoglobulins bind to the specific epitope, **B cell activated**
  - o Activated B cell undergoes **clonal expansion (proliferation)**
  - o B cell usually requires **assistance of a T helper cell (T$_H$)**
  - o Antigen needing a **T$_H$ cell** for antibody production called a **T-dependent antigen** (mainly proteins found on: viruses, bacteria, foreign red blood cells, and hapten with their carriers)
    - ■ For antibodies to be produced, in response to a **T-dependent antigen,** both B and T cells be must be activated and interact
    - ■ **B cells contact the antigen** (the antigen contacts the surface immunoglobulins on the B cell and the **antigen is enzymatically processed within the B cell**)
    - ■ The **fragment** processed combines with the **major histocompatibility complex (MHC)**
    - ■ **MHC** (a collection of genes that encode molecules of glycoproteins), found on plasma membrane on mammalian nucleated cells; **in humans, MHC** known as **human leukocyte antigen (HLA) System**
      - ✓ **FYI: MHC are cell surface markers divided into three classes: I, II, III**
    - ■ The **antigenic fragment and the MHC** are displayed on the B cell's surface, for receptors on the **T helper cell to identify**
    - ■ The **MHC** is of **class II**: found only on the surface of **antigen presenting cells (APC's), B cell**
    - ■ The **T$_H$ cell** in contact with the antigenic fragment, presented on the B cell, **becomes activated and produces cytokines**
    - ■ **Cytokines** deliver a message causing **activation of the B cell**
    - ■ **B cell proliferates** into a large **clone of cells**
    - ■ **These clones** can proliferate into **antibody producing plasma cells or memory cells**
      - ✓ **Clonal selection**: Each B cell recognizes only one type of antigen. An encounter with a particular antigen triggers proliferation of a B cell, to proliferate a clone of cells that is specific for that antigen
  - o First class of antibodies detected in the primary response is IgM
  - o Individual B cell can make different classes of antibodies (IgG, IgE, or IgA); termed **class switching**; when IgG begins to be produced, production of IgM will cease
  - o **Clonal deletion**: B cells which may cause harm to host tissue or self, usually eliminated at the immature lymphocyte stage
  - o **Antigens that stimulate B cells directly without help from T cells called T-independent antigens**
    - ■ Have repeating subunits like those found in polysaccharides or lipopolysaccharides
    - ■ Repeating units bind to multiple B cell receptors

- ■ **T-independent antigens** provoke a weaker immune response; composed primarily of IgM and no memory cells
- ■ Example: bacterial capsules
- ● **The Diversity of Antibodies**
  - o Human immune system can recognize an incredible amount of antigens
  - o Recombination of genes occurs in embryonic B cells; this causes mature B cells, each to have different genes for the V region of their antibodies

F. Antigen-Antibody Binding and its Results
- ● An **antigen-antibody complex** forms when an antibody attaches to its specific **epitope** (or **antigenic determinant**) on an antigen
- ● **Affinity**: is the strength of the bond between antigen and antibody; the closer the fit, the higher the affinity and vice versa
- ● **Specificity**: ability to distinguish between minor differences in the aa sequence of a protein
- ● Removal of infectious agents and toxins from the body is accomplished by a few mechanisms
  - o **Agglutination**: antibodies **clump together** antigens making them easy to be ingested by phagocytes
  - o **Opsonization: antibody coats the antigen** making it easier for phagocytic cells to ingest and lyse
  - o **Neutralization: IgG** antibodies **blocks antigens** (microbes or toxins) from attaching to targeted cell
  - o **Antibody-dependent cell-mediated cytotoxicity:** target cell/organism coated with antibodies; destruction of target cell/organism by macrophages, eosinophils, NK cells
  - o **Activation of complement:** used when infectious agents are coated with reactive proteins which cause IgG and IgM antibodies to attach to the agent→lyses of cell membrane

G. T Cells and Cellular Immunity
- ● **T cells** response to bacteria, parasites, viruses which **invade and live within cells (intracellular pathogens)**
- ● Develop from stem cells in bone marrow and **migrate to the thymus gland** where they mature, then to the lymphatic system
- ● **Thymic selection: thymus** removes most **immatureT cells** that do not recognize MHC-self molecules
- ● In late adulthood, the ability to create **T cells** diminishes→weaker immune system
- ● **T cells recognition of an antigen** requires the antigen first **be processed** by specialized **antigen-presenting cells (APC's)**, such as macrophages and dendritic cells
- ● The antigen is ingested by the APC; an **antigenic fragment** is presented on the surface of the cell together with a **MHC molecule**
- ● **Classes of T Cells**
  - o There are classes of **T cells** that are **based on different functions**
    - ■ **T helper cells:** cooperate with B cells in the production of antibodies (through cytokine signaling); interact more directly with antigens
    - ■ Two populations of **T cells**
      - ✓ **T helper cells (T_H):** recognize antigen presented on macrophages and activate the macrophage
      - ✓ **T cytotoxic cells (T_C):** can differentiate into an effector cell called **cytotoxic T lymphocytes (CTL)**
  - o **T cells** also classified by certain glycoproteins on their surface called **clusters of differentiation (CD)**
    - ■ **CD:** important for adhesion to receptors

   ✓ **CD4$^+$**: include **T$_H$ cells**; bind to MHC class II molecules on B cells and APCs

   ✓ **CD8$^+$**: include **T$_C$ cells**; bind to MHC class I molecules

- **T Helper Cells (CD4$^+$ T Cells)**
  - To be activated, an **APC/dendritic cell ingests an antigen** (microbe)
  - The antigen is processed into antigenic fragments; the fragments combine with MHC class II molecules and are displayed on APC surface
  - **Signal one: TCR (T cell receptor)** recognizes/binds to the MHC-antigen complex; **Signal two: APC is stimulated to secrete a costimulatory molecule**
  - **These two signals activate the T$_H$ cell to produce cytokines**
  - Cytokines cause the **T$_H$ cell** to become activated
  - Activated **T$_H$ cell** begins to proliferate
  - Proliferating **T$_H$ cells** differentiate into **populations of subsets**
    - **T$_H$1**: activate cells involved in **cellular immunity**; control of intracellular pathogens; delayed hypersensitivity reactions; stimulates macrophages
    - **T$_H$2**: associated with **allergic reactions and parasitic infections**; production of **IgE**
    - **T$_H$17**: activate **innate immunity and responds to extracellular bacteria and fungi**; recruits neutrophils; produce large amounts of cytokine **IL-17**
    - **T$_{FH}$ (follicular helper T cells)**: stimulate B cells to produce plasma cells
- **T Regulatory Cells (T$_{reg}$)**
  - Formally called **T suppressor cells**; suppress **T cells** against self
  - Carry an additional **CD25 molecule**
- **T Cytotoxic Cells (CD8$^+$ T Cells)**
  - Precursors to **CTLs**
  - Carry fragments of **endogenous antigens** (generally synthesized within the cell; mostly viral or parasitic in origin)
  - Other target cells are tumor cells and transplanted foreign tissue
  - **Activated by endogenous antigens and MHC class I on a target cell** and transformed into CTL
  - CTLs lyse target cells by releasing a pore-forming protein, **perforin** and induce **apoptosis**

H. Antigen-Presenting Cells (APCs)

- Include other forms of B cells, dendritic cells, and macrophages
  - **Dendritic Cells**
    - The **primary APCs** to induce immune responses to T cells
    - Have long extensions called dendrites
    - In skin and genital tract (called **Langerhans cells**), lymph nodes, spleen, thymus
  - **Macrophages**
    - Important for innate immunity and ridding the body of old worn out blood cells, cellular remnants, debris
    - Usually in resting state, until stimulated (by ingesting antigenic material, cytokines)
    - Once stimulated they become more effective as APCs and phagocytes
- **APCs** migrate from their location to lymph nodes or lymphoid tissues, **after taking up an antigen**
  - They present the antigen to T cells in lymph nodes or lymphoid tissues

I. Extracellular Killing by the Immune System

- **Natural killer (NK) cells**: destroy certain virus-infected cells and tumor cells; attacks parasites
- **NK cells** don't need to be stimulated by an antigen; they first contact the target cell and determine if it expresses MHC self-antigens. If it does not, **NK cells** will kill the target cell by mechanisms similar to **CTL**; forms pores in target cell→ lysis or apoptosis; **antibody-dependent cell-mediated cytotoxicity**

J. Antibody-Dependent Cell Mediated Cytotoxicity (ADCC)
- **NK and macrophages:** able to lyse antibody-coated cells (protozoa, helminthes)

K. Cytokines: Chemical Messengers of Immune Cells
- **Cytokines:** chemicals messengers in which the cells of the immune system communicate
- Soluble proteins or glycoproteins produced by practically all cells of the immune system in response to a stimulus
- Examples include
  - **Interleukins (IL-1, and so on):** serve as communicators between leukocytes
  - **Chemokines:** cause leukocytes to move to the site of infection
  - **Interferons(IFN-α, and so on):** protect cells from viral infections
  - **Tumor necrosis factor (TNF-α, and so on):** promotes the inflammatory reaction
  - **Hematopoietic cytokines (IL-3, and so on; colony stimulating factors (CSFs)):** promote the development of white blood cells
- Over production can lead to tissue damage: **cytokine storm**

L. Immunological Memory
- **Antibody titer:** relative amount of antibody in the serum; help identify intensity of the antibody-mediated humoral response
- **Pattern of primary response to an antigen**
  - After initial contact with antigen, no detectable antibodies for 4 to 7 days
  - Then, slow rise in titer: **first IgM** antibodies produced **followed, by IgG** peaking in 10 to 17 days
  - This is followed by antibody titer gradually declining
- **Pattern of Secondary (memory or anamnestic) response**
  - After second exposure to same antigen, memory cells stimulated (formed at initial exposure) to rapidly produce large amounts of antibody; rapidly reaching a peak in 2 to 7 days, lasting more days, and of greater magnitude
  - Antibodies produced are **mostly IgG**
- Similar response occurs with **T cells**, which is important in establishing lifelong memory for distinguishing self from nonself

MICROBIOLOGY

PRACTICAL APPLICATIONS of IMMUNOLOGY

A. Vaccines
- Variolation: an early form of **vaccination**
- **Edward Jenner** and the "dairy maid" cowpox; injected cowpox to protect from smallpox
- **Vaccine:** suspension or fraction of organisms used to induce an immune response
- **Principles and Effects of Vaccination**
  - **Jenner's injections'** (via skin scratch) **provoked a primary immune response leading to the formation of antibodies and long term memory cells**
  - The memory cells →secondary immune response
  - Controlling a disease does not necessarily require everyone be immune to it
  - If most of population immune, one can get **"herd immunity": sporadic cases** occur due to **small numbers of susceptible individuals to support the spread**
  - Many vaccines in the United States
    - Childhood immunizations
    - Travelers, college freshmen, elderly, health care providers, females, military

B. Types of Vaccines and their Characteristics
- **Live Attenuated Vaccines**
  - **Living, but weakened** microorganisms
  - Live attenuated vaccines closely mimic an actual infection → lifelong immunity achieved; achieved without booster immunization
  - **Disadvantage:** the live microbes can back mutate to a virulent form
  - **Not recommended for immunocompromised persons**
  - **Diseases:** MMR, chicken pox, Herpes zoster, influenza (nasal administration)
- **Inactivated Killed Vaccines**
  - Use **microbes that have been killed:** by formalin, phenol
  - Considered safer that live attenuated vaccines
  - Often require repeated booster
  - **Diseases:** rabies, influenza, Salk polio, bacterial vaccines (pneumococcal pneumonia and cholera), pertussi, typhoid
- **Subunit Vaccines**
  - **Use antigenic fragments** of the microbe **which best stimulate an immune response**
    - **Recombinant vaccines: vaccines produced by genetic engineering techniques**; produce the desired antigenic fragment
      - ✓ Hepatitis B virus
    - **Toxoids (Inactivated toxins):** vaccines which are **directed at toxins produced by the pathogen**
      - ✓ Usually require series of injections for full immunity, followed by boosters Q 10 years
      - ✓ Tetanus and diptheria toxoids
  - Safer vaccines because they cannot reproduce in the recipient; they contain little or no extraneous material→ less side effects
- **Conjugated Vaccines**
  - Used in dealing with children who develop weak/poor immune responses to vaccines **based on "capsular polysaccharides"**

116

- o These **"polysaccharides"** are **T-independent antigens**
- o Child's immune system does not respond well to these antigens until age 15-24 months
- o These **'polysaccharides'** are **combined with proteins** such as diptheria or tetanus toxoid
  - ■ *Haemophilus influenzae* type b: protects at two months of age
- **Nucleic acid (DNA) Vaccines**
  - o **Animal experiments** show **plasmids of "naked" DNA** injected into muscle →production of **the antigenic proteins encoded in the DNA**
  - o These **antigenic proteins** carried to red bone marrow; persist and stimulate humoral and cellular immune responses
  - o Two DNA vaccines **for animals** are approved
    - ■ One protects horses from West Nile Virus
    - ■ One protects salmon from a viral disease
  - o **Clinical test in humans underway**
- **The Development of New Vaccines**
  - o Vaccine developments targeted at
    - ■ Not only preventing the disease, but prevent it from ever occurring again
    - ■ Swallowed (oral), injected, applied as a patch, and administered once in a lifetime
    - ■ Affordable
    - ■ Be developed on animal, plant, and humans cell cultures
    - ■ Developing vaccines which do not grow well in cell cultures (recombinant vaccines and DNA vaccines)
    - ■ Decrease fear of litigations and liability of vaccine manufacturers
    - ■ Remain stable without refrigeration
    - ■ Developing vaccines that grant T cell immunity (tuberculosis, HIV, cancer)
    - ■ Antigenic variability (changing annually requiring a new vaccine)
    - ■ Potentials for treating addictions (drugs), cancer
- **Adjuvants**
  - o Chemical additives used to improve the effectiveness of vaccines
  - o **Certain aluminum salts, when combined with many vaccines, improve vaccines effectiveness**
    - ■ **Alum:** the only adjuvant approved for **use in humans in the United States**
  - o Mechanism as to how **adjuvants** work is not known in detail
- **Safety of Vaccines**
  - o Vaccines still remain the safest and most effective means of preventing infectious disease in children
  - o No vaccine will ever be perfectly safe or perfectly effective

C. Diagnostic Immunology
- **Essential to diagnostic tests are sensitivity and specificity**
  - o **Sensitivity:** the percentage of positive samples the test correctly detects [(TP/(TP+FN)x100]
  - o **Specificity:** determined by the percentage of false positive results the test gives [(TN/TN+FP) x100]
- **Immunologic-Based Diagnostic Tests**
  - o One of the first diagnostic tests: **Robert Koch (against tuberculosis)**
    - ■ Guinea pigs injected with suspension of *Mycobacterium tuberculosis*→ injection site red/ swollen 1-2 days later (a **positive result** for the tuberculin skin test)
  - o Many diagnostic tests based on interactions of humoral antibodies with antigens
    - ■ A **known antibody** can be used to identify an **unknown antigen**, and a **known antigen** can be used to identify an **unknown antibody**
- **Monoclonal Antibodies**
  - o **B cells** a potential source of a single type of antibody

- o Isolation and cultivation of B cells producing a single type of antibody in unlimited supply technique used
  - Using **myelomas** (cancerous B cells which are isolated and propagated indefinitely) and **hybridomas** (fused "cancer" B cell with antibody-producing normal B cell)
- o **Hybridomas**: produce genetically identical cells which produce antibodies characteristic of the ancestral B cell
  - These identical antibody molecules called **monoclonal antibodies,** or **Mabs**
- o **Mabs** used as diagnostic tools: recognize certain bacterial pathogens; pregnancy test; class of drugs (treatment for multiple sclerosis, cancer, asthma, etc..); rheumatoid arthritis (Remicade)
- o **Chimeric monoclonal antibodies:** use genetically modified mice to make a **human-murine hybrid**
  - Variable part of antibody, including antigen-binding site: murine; Constant region: human source
  - These **Mabs** about 66% human
  - Example: rituximab
- o **Humanized antibodies:** murine portion limited to antigen-binding sites
  - **Mabs** about 90% human
  - Example: alemutuzumab
- o **Fully human antibodies:** eventual goal; fully human antibodies
- **Precipitation Reactions:** involve the reaction of **soluble antigens with IgG or IgM** antibodies forming large interlocking molecules called **lattices**
  - o Occurs in **two stages**
    - Antigens and antibodies form antigen-antibody complexes (**fast reaction**)
    - Then, antigen-antibody complex form lattices that precipitate (**slow reaction**)
      - ✓ Reaction occurs only when ratio of antigen to antibody is optimal; will see **"cloudy line"** of precipitation at the zone of equivalence (called **precipitin ring test**)
  - o Examples
    - **Immunodiffusion tests:** precipitation reaction carried out in an agar gel medium (in a Petri plate or glass slide); line of visible precipitate develops between the wells
    - **Electrophoresis:** speeds up movement of antigen and antibody; using electrodes
    - **Immunoelectrophoresis: electrophoresis with immunodiffusion**
      - ✓ **Western blot test:** AIDS testing
- **Agglutination Reactions:** involve either **particulate antigens** (particles such as cells which carry antigenic molecules) **or soluble antigens adhering to particles**
  - o These antigens are linked together by antibodies to form visible aggregates
  - o Very sensitive, easy to read
  - o Classified as **either direct or indirect**
    - <u>**Direct agglutination test (DAT)**</u>: detect **antibodies against cellular antigens** (RBC's, bacteria, fungi)
      - ✓ **Patient's serum** (unknown **antibody**); combine with **known antigen** in a microtiter plate (has wells)
      - ✓ **Amount of antigen in a well is the same**; **serum** containing antibodies **is diluted**
      - ✓ *Titer*: **the concentration of serum antibody;** the higher the serum antibody titer, the greater the immunity to the disease
      - ✓ *Titer alone*: **of limited use** in diagnosing existing illness
      - ✓ *Rise in titer*: significant; higher later in disease course, than onset
      - ✓ *Seroconversion*: patients' blood had **no antibody before** the illness, but a significant rising *titer* while the disease is progressing, this change is diagnostic; example: HIV infections

- **Indirect (Passive) agglutination test (IAT):** using **particles coated with antigens** (antigens are **absorbed onto particles** like bentonite clay, **latex spheres**)to detect **antibodies**
  - ✓ Antibody reacts with the soluble antigen adhering to the particles
  - ✓ The **particles agglutinate with one another**
  - ✓ Same principle can be applied in reverse: using **particles coated with antibodies** to detect **antigens**
  - ✓ Very rapid results
- **Hemagglutination:** agglutination reactions involving **the clumping of RBC's**
  - ✓ Test involves **RBC surface antigens** and **their complimentary antibodies**
  - ✓ Used in **blood typing**; diagnosing infectious mononucleosis
- **Viral hemagglutination:** certain viruses **agglutinate RBC's without antigen-antibody reaction**
  - ✓ Reaction inhibited by antibodies that neutralize the agglutinating virus
  - ✓ Viruses: mumps, measles, influenza
- **Neutralization Reactions**
  - o Antigen-antibody reaction in which **the harmful effects of a bacterial exotoxin or virus are blocked by specific antibodies**
  - o This **neutralizing substance** called **antitoxin**; it is a **specific antibody produced by the host** as it responds to a bacterial exotoxin or toxoid
  - o **Antitoxin** combines with the exotoxin to neutralize it
  - o **Antitoxins** produced in an animal injected into humans to produce passive immunity
    - Examples: antitoxins from horses to treat diphtheria, botulism; antitoxin from human origin to treat tetanus
  - o Used as diagnostic tests
    - **Vitro neutralization test:** knowing certain viruses exhibit certain cytopathic effects in cell cultures or embryonated eggs, test can be used to detect the presence of neutralizing viral antibodies; **test very complex**
    - **Viral hemagglutination inhibition test:** certain viruses **agglutinate RBC's;** if serum contains antibodies against these viruses, these antibodies will react with viruses and neutralize them
      - ✓ Used in diagnosing: influenza, mumps, measles, other virus causing infections
- **Complement-Fixation Reactions**
  - o **Complement:** a group of serum proteins
  - o **Complement** binds to the antigen-antibody complex during most antigen-antibody reactions, and is used up; process called **complement fixation**
  - o Used to detect **small amounts of antibody**
  - o Syphilis (Wassermann test), certain viral, fungal, rickettsial diseases
  - o Performed in two stages: **complement-fixation** and **indicator**
- **Flourescent-Antibody (FA) Techniques**
  - o **Identify microbes** and **detect the presence of a specific antibody** in serum
  - o Combine **fluorescent dyes with antibodies** to make them fluoresce when exposed to UV light
  - o Techniques are quick, sensitive, very specific
  - o Example: Rabies
  - o Two types: **Direct and Indirect**
    - **Direct FA tests:** used to **identify a microbe** in a clinical specimen
      - ✓ Specimen containing the antigen is fixed on a slide
      - ✓ **Fluorescein-labeled antibodies added**→ slide incubated→slide is washed→ examined under fluorescence microscope for **yellow-green fluorescence**

- **Indirect FA tests:** used to **detect** the presence of **a specific antibody** in the serum following exposure to a microbe; more sensitive than the direct tests
  - ✓ Known antigen is fixed to a slide; test serum (with antibodies) added
  - ✓ If antibody that is specific to the microbe is present, will form a complex
  - ✓ **Fluorescein-labeled anti-human immune serum globulin (anti-HISG) added to slide to make complex visible**
  - ✓ Anti-HISG present only if the specific antibody has reacted with its antigen
  - ✓ Slide incubated →rinsed→ examined under fluorescence microscope
  - ✓ **If known antigen fixed on slide fluoresces, antibody specific to the test antigen is present**
  - o **Fluorescence-activated cell sorter (FACS):** adaptation of fluorescent antibodies; a modified flow cytometer
    - Used to detect and separate different classes of cells labeled with antibodies
      - ✓ Follow the progression of AIDS, by counting **CD4⁺ T cells**

- **Enzyme-Linked Immunosorbent Assay (ELISA)**
  - o Uses **antibodies linked to an enzyme (horseradish peroxidase or alkaline phosphatase)**
  - o **Two methods: Direct and Indirect;** both use microtiter plates
    - **Direct ELISA:** detects antigens
      - ✓ **Specific antibodies** absorbed to well
      - ✓ Sample (contains unidentified **antigen**) added; **antigen-antibody complex** formed
      - ✓ An **enzyme-linked antibody (specific for test antigen)** added
      - ✓ **If "absorbed antibody" and "known specific antigen" bind,** forms a **sandwich** (antigen between two antibodies)
      - ✓ Reaction visible due to enzyme linked to a **substrate** unbound enzyme-linked antibody washed
      - ✓ Used to detect drugs in urine
    - **Indirect ELISA:** detects antibodies
      - ✓ **Specific antigens** (from lab) absorbed to well
      - ✓ **Antiserum (contains antibodies)** added; **antigen-antibody complex** formed
      - ✓ **Enzyme-linked anti-HISG (an Ig that attaches to any antibody) is added;** binds to the complex; forms a **sandwich**
      - ✓ Color **substrate added→visibility**
      - ✓ Used to screen blood for antibodies to HIV

- **Western Blotting (Immunoblotting)**
  - o Identifies a **specific protein** in a mixture
  - o Example: **identifying a specific antibody** in a mixture
    - **Components** in mixture separated by **electrophoresis** in a gel; transferred to a **protein-binding sheet (blotter)**
    - **Blotter** (containing protein/antigen) flooded with an **enzyme-linked antibody;** location of the **antigen and enzyme-linked** antibody reactant visualized using a color-reacting label
    - Confirmatory test for HIV infection

F. The Future of Diagnostic and Therapeutic Immunology
- **Monoclonal antibodies** have made new diagnostic testing possible
- It is possible to make large, inexpensive amounts of specific antibodies
- Test are more sensitive, specific, rapid, and simpler to perform
- Nonimmunological test like **PCR** and **DNA probes** are increasing in usage (automated)
- Tests could possibly be directed at preventing diseases

MICROBIOLOGY

DISORDERS ASSOCIATED with the IMMUNE SYSTEM

A. Introduction
- The reactions of the immune system can also produce harmful results
- The immune system can 'fail' causing infections and/or immunosuppression
- Certain antigens called 'super antigens' can cause adverse host responses

B. Hypersensitivity
- Also termed **"allergy" is an antigenic response beyond normal**
- Occurs in person **previously sensitized** to an **allergen (antigen)**; exposed to **antigen again**; immune system reacts to **antigen** in a damaging way
- **Four principle types of hypersensitivity reactions**
  - **Type I (Anaphylactic) Reactions**
    - **Anaphylactic:** means the opposite of protected
    - Occurs within **2 to 30 mins** after reexposure
    - **IgE mediated reaction:** IgE antibodies produced in response to antigen
      - ✓ **IgE binds to mast cells or basophils**
      - ✓ Binding of two adjacent **IgE antibodies to the antigen** causes **degranulation** (release of **substances** like histamine, leukotrienes, prostaglandins)
      - ✓ These '**substances**' cause: edema (swelling), erythema (redness), increased mucus secretion, bronchial spasms
    - **Systemic Anaphylaxis (aka Anaphylactic Shock)**
      - ✓ **Injected antigens** more likely to cause dramatic response
      - ✓ Results in rapid drop in BP, bronchospasms→death within a few minutes
      - ✓ Treatment with epinephrine
      - ✓ Example: penicillin
    - **Localized Anaphylaxis**
      - ✓ Caused by **ingested** (milk, fish, sulfites, certain foods) **or inhaled** (pollen) **antigens** entering body
      - ✓ Symptoms: allergic rhinitis, asthma, diarrhea
    - **Prevention of Anaphylactic Reactions:** avoid contact; skin tests: sensitivity to allergen indicated by rapid inflammatory reaction (redness, swelling, pain, heat) at inoculation site; undergo **desensitization**
  - **Type II (Cytotoxic) Reactions**
    - Involves the **activation of complement** (serum proteins) **by the combination of IgG or IgM** antibodies with an **'antigenic cell'** leading to **lysis of the cell**
    - Onset within **5 to 12 hrs**
    - **Transfusion reactions** (red blood cells destroyed) most common type
    - **ABO Blood Group System**
      - ✓ Four principle types based on the presence or absence of **carbohydrate antigens on RBC walls (AB, A, B, O)**
      - ✓ Natural **antibodies** against the '**opposite**' antigen exist in the serum
      - ✓ Incompatible blood transfusions→ RBC lyses
        - ❖ If type 'A' blood transfused (mixed) with A, or O blood, can transfuse; **no lysis**

❖ If type 'A' blood transfused (mixed) with B Blood→transfusion causes **lysis**

- **Rh Blood Group System**
  - ✓ Different surface antigen, **called 'Rh factor'** on RBC walls
  - ✓ **85% of the population** with this antigen designated **Rh⁺**
  - ✓ Remaining designated **Rh⁻ ; absence of Rh factor** can lead to sensitization upon exposure
  - ✓ Antibodies that react with the **Rh⁺** do not occur naturally in the serum of **Rh⁻** individuals
    - ❖ Exposure to this antigen (**Rh⁺**) can lead to sensitization producing **anti-Rh antibodies**
- **Blood Transfusions and Rh Incompatibility**
  - ✓ When **Rh⁻** person receives **Rh⁺**blood, **Rh⁻** person stimulates production of **anti-Rh antibodies**
  - ✓ If **Rh⁻** person subsequently exposed to **Rh⁺ blood, hemolysis will occur**
- **Hemolytic Disease of the Newborn (HDNB)**
  - ✓ An **Rh⁻** woman and an **Rh⁺** man produce a child; if child is **Rh⁺**, **Rh⁻** mother can become sensitized (fetal **Rh⁺ RBC's** enter maternal circulation, mother produces **anti-Rh antibodies**); if subsequent pregnancy is **Rh⁺**, maternal **anti-Rh antibodies** cross placenta **destroying fetal RBC's**
  - ✓ **HDNB:** prevented by passive immunization (**RhoGAM**); fetal transfusion
- **Drug-Induced Cytotoxic Reactions**
  - ✓ **Thrombocytopenia purpuria: thrombocytes** coated with a **drug molecule** (example is **quinine,** considered a **hapten**) become antigenic; both antibody and complement needed for **thrombocyte lysis**
  - ○ **Type III (Immune Complex) Reactions**
    - Usually involves **IgG antibodies** and **antigens** circulating in the **serum** forming complexes which **deposit** causing inflammatory damage in organs
    - Occurs when a certain **antigen-antibody complex** ratio exists, with slight **excess of antigen;** these **complexes circulate** in blood, pass between cells of blood vessels and **become trapped; trapped complex** activates complement and attracts inflammatory cells→damage to endothelial cells basement membrane
    - Damage occurs within **2 to 8 hrs**
    - Example: **Glomerulonephritis**
  - ○ **Type IV (Delayed Cell-Mediated) Reactions**
    - Caused mainly by **T cells**
    - Sensitized individual is exposed, again, to an antigen causing a **delayed hypersensitivity reaction**
    - **Delay** due to time it takes participating **T cells** and **macrophages** to migrate to site of **foreign antigens**
    - Occurs within **24 to 48 hrs**
    - **Causes of Delayed Cell-Mediated Reactions**: foreign **antigens** phagocytized by macrophages, then **presented to T cell** surface; causes **T cell to proliferate** into **mature differentiated T cells** and memory cells; if sensitized person **reexposed to same antigen, memory cells activate T cells** (release cytokines) in their interaction with the target antigen
    - **Delayed Cell-Mediated Hypersensitivity Reactions of the Skin**
      - ✓ *Mycobacterium tuberculosis:* often located in macrophages; organism **can stimulate a delayed cell-mediated immune response**
        - ❖ As a screening test, **protein components** of the bacteria **injected into skin**
        - ❖ If recipient has (or has had) previous infection→**induration and reddening** at site in 24 to 48 hours

    ✓ **Allergic contact dermatitis:** usually caused by **haptens** which **combine with proteins in the skin**→ **immune response**

       ❖ Examples: latex, makeup, metals, poison ivy, jewelry

C. Autoimmune Diseases

- Occurs when the **immune system is unable to discriminate self from non-self;** loss of **self-tolerance**
- Greater than **40 autoimmune diseases** identified
- Leads to the **production of antibodies against one's own body**
- Autoimmune reactions can be: **cytotoxic, immune complex, cell-mediated**
  - o **Cytotoxic Autoimmune Reactions**
    - ■ **Antibodies react to cell-surface antigens, but no cytotoxic destruction of the cells**
      - ✓ **Graves' disease:** thyroid gland stimulated to produce large amounts of thyroid hormones; **abnormal antibodies released that mimic TSH**; thyroid gland now producing excessive amount of hormones causing: pounding heart, trembling, sweating; **goiter**
      - ✓ **Myasthenia gravis:** caused by **antibodies coating acetylcholine receptors;** causes inability of nerve impulses to reach muscles causing progressive muscle weakness; can lead to respiratory arrest
  - o **Immune Complex Autoimmune Reactions**
    - ■ **Deposition of immune complexes leads to tissue damage**
      - ✓ **Rheumatoid arthritis:** caused by immune **complexes of IgM, IgG, and complement** which **deposit in joints;** leads to chronic inflammation and damage to cartilage and bone of the joint; **immune complexes** called **rheumatoid factors** may be formed by **IgM binding** normal **IgG**
      - ✓ **Systemic lupus erythematosus:** a systemic **autoimmune disease;** involves **immune complex reactions** mainly affecting women; etiology not well understood; individual produces **antibodies** directed **at parts of their own cells, including DNA;** affects kidney glomeruli
  - o **Cell-Mediated Autoimmune Reactions**
    - ■ **Destruction of cells mediated by T-cells**
      - ✓ **Multiple sclerosis: T cells and macrophages attack myelin sheath** of nerves; progressive disease causing fatigue, weakness, paralysis; etiology unknown (? Infective agent)
      - ✓ **Insulin-dependent diabetes mellitus:** causes by **destruction of insulin-secreting cells of the pancreas**
      - ✓ **Psoriasis:** considered to be a $T_H 1$ disease; symptoms are itchy-red patches of thickened skin; may develop into **psoriatic arthritis**

D. Reactions Related to the Human Leukocyte Antigen (HLA) Complex

- Genetic characteristics of individuals also expressed in the composition of the **self-molecules on one's cell surfaces** (some of these self-molecules **called histocompatibility antigens**)
- Genes controlling the production of these molecules known as the **major histocompatibility complex (MHC);** in humans, these genes called **humans leukocyte antigen (HLA) complex**
- **HLA typing:** a method used to identify and compare **HLAs**
- Certain **HLAs related to** increased susceptibility to certain diseases
- **HLA typing:** used in **transplant surgery;** donor and recipient must be matched by **tissue typing;** to **prevent rejection** of transplant, **HLA and ABO blood group antigens matched** as closely as possible

- **Serological tissue typing technique:** lymphocytes (recipient) incubated with standardized monoclonal antibodies (selected specific antiserum) that are specific for particular HLA's; complement and dye added; cell damaged by complement take up dye; this positive result indicates the person (recipient) has the particular HLA being tested for
- **Polymerase chain reaction (PCR):** a more accurate technique for analyzing **HLA;** amplifies **donor and recipients DNA**
  - o **Reactions to Transplantation:** transplants **recognized as foreign are rejected** (are attacked by T cells, activated macrophages, or antibodies); some transplants or grafts **do not stimulate an immune response**
    - **Privileged sites:** antibodies do not circulate in that area (**cornea, brain**)
    - **Privileged tissues:** does not stimulate an immune response (**human heart valve with pig valve; pregnancy**)
    - **Stem Cells:** cells capable of generating any of the cell types making up the body
      - ✓ Specifically **embryonic stem cells (ESCs):** pluripotent
      - ✓ Adult stem cells (ASCs): produce few different cell types
      - ✓ Induced pluripotent stem cells (**iPSCs**): genetically reprogrammed ASCs by using viruses
      - ✓ Hematopoietic stem cells (**HPSc**): umbilical cord blood cells
    - **Grafts: based on genetic makeup**
      - ✓ **Autograft: self to self**; own tissue grafted to another part of body; not rejected (**burn victim**)
      - ✓ **Isograft: identical twins**; same genetic makeup; not rejected (**kidney**)
      - ✓ **Allografts: blood relatives, siblings**; immune response triggered; attempts to closely match the HLAs to reduce rejection
      - ✓ **Xenotransplantation products** (formerly called **Xenograft**): tissue or organs transplanted from **animals;** severe immune response (**pig heart valves**)
      - ✓ **Hyperacute rejection:** caused by development of antibodies against transplanted tissue: (example: **kidney transplant**); these antibodies, with the help of complement, attack the transplant tissue and destroy it within an hour
    - **Bone Marrow Transplants (also known as hematopoietic stem cell transplants)**
      - ✓ Bone marrow stem cells give rise to RBC's and immune system lymphocytes
      - ✓ Usually done for individuals who lack the ability to produce B cells and T cells, or who suffer from leukemia
      - ✓ Goal: to enable recipient to produce such normal cells
      - ✓ Can result in **graft-versus-host (GVH) disease:** when transplanted marrow contains immunocompetent cells, a cell- mediated immune response against the tissue in which it has been transplanted, can occur; can be fatal
      - ✓ Instead of the **Bone marrow transplant technique, umbilical cord blood (UCB) used**
      - ✓ **UCB:** rich in stem cells; less risk of GVH disease

E. Immunosuppression
- In order to **prevent "transplant rejection"**, recipients usually receive some form of an **Immunosuppressant** to suppress **"normal" immune response**
- **Cell-mediated immunity first and most important to suppress**
- Immunosuppressive agents usually administered in combinations
  - o **Cyclosporine** (from a mold): **suppresses secretion of interleukin-2 (IL-2),** disrupting cell-mediated immunity by cytotoxic T cells; serious side effects; has little effect in antibody production by the humoral immune system
  - o **Tacrolimus** (FK506): **similar to cyclosporine**
  - o **Sirolimus** (Rapamune): **inhibits both cell-mediated** and **humoral immunity;** used in stents

- o **Mycophenolate: inhibits proliferation of T and B cells**
- o **Basiliximab and Daclizuma:** (chimeric antibodies) **block IL-2**

F. Immunodeficiency's
- **Immunodeficiency:** is the absence of a sufficient immune response
- **Either Congenital or Acquired**
  - o **Congenital:** born with a defective immune system; absent or defective inherited gene (s)
    - ✓ **DiGeorge syndrome:** do not have a **thymus gland; do not produce T cells;** lack cell-mediated immunity
  - o **Acquired:** due to drugs, infectious agents, cancer (Hodgkin's), AIDS

G. The Immune System and Cancer
- A normal cell becomes **cancerous when it undergoes transformation and proliferates uncontrollably**
- The **surface of tumor cells** acquire **tumor-associated antigens**; marks them as nonself causing **T cells** to become activated; leads to lysis of cancer cells (individual cancer cells that arise are attacked by the immune system)
- In some cases, **no antigenic marker** for immune system to attack; **tumor cells** can **reproduce rapidly**, exceeding a response of the immune system; **tumor cells** can **attach to tissue and become vascularized** becoming invisible to the immune system

H. Immunotherapy for Cancer
- **The treatment of cancer via immunological means**
- **Known endotoxins** from certain bacteria **stimulate** the production of **tumor necrosis factor (TNF)** by macrophages; TNF interferes with blood supply of cancers in animals
- In animals, when injected with dead tumor cells (as a vaccine), did not develop tumors when injected with live cells from these tumors
- **Cancer vaccines:** might be **therapeutic** (used to treat existing cancers) or **prophylactic** (to prevent the development of cancer)
  - o **Therapeutic cancer vaccines:** for advanced prostate cancer
  - o **Prophylactic cancer vaccines: hepatitis B virus** (liver cancer); **Gardasil** (cervical cancer)
- Monoclonal antibodies: promising tools for delivering cancer treatment
  - o **Herceptin:** used in breast cancer treatment; neutralizes **HER2 (determined growth factor)** that promotes proliferation of cancer cells
  - o **Immunotoxins** (a monoclonal antibody *and* toxic agent) used: specifically targets and kills the tumor cells with little damage to normal healthy cells
- **Neutralize cytokines** causing decreased blood supply to tumor cell proliferation
- Creating vaccines against cancers: **Marek's disease in poultry**

I. Acquired Immunodeficiency Syndrome (AIDS)
- A cluster of cases of *Pneumocystis* pneumonia appeared in Los Angeles area, in 1981; associated with rare skin and blood vessel disease (**Kaposi's sarcoma**)
- **Young homosexual males mainly** affected; showing loss of immune function caused by **a virus** which selectively infects **helper T cells; virus** now known as human immunodeficiency virus (**HIV**)
  - o **Origins of AIDS**
    - ■ ? arisen from mutation of a virus originally endemic to central areas of Africa
    - ■ Benign virus originally infected monkeys and chimpanzees

- **HIV-2** (type of HIV that is weakly contagious) is a mutation of a simian immunodeficiency virus (SIV) carried by monkeys; **HIV-1** genetically related to another SIV carried by chimpanzees in central Africa; later **infected humans**
- Colonization→urbanization→transportation→spread
- Earliest documented case in 1959 (Belgian Congo)
- Western world, case of AIDS via death of a Norwegian sailor in 1976

o **HIV Infection**
  - **The Structure of HIV**
    - ✓ Of the genus *Lentivirus*; **a retrovirus**
    - ✓ Consist of: two identical strands of **RNA,** enzyme **reverse transcriptase,** an **envelope** of phospholipids; **envelop** has **glycoprotein spikes (termed gp120)**
  - **Infectiveness and Pathogenicity of HIV**
    - ✓ **HIV** spread by dendritic cells
    - ✓ **HIV** goes through steps of attachment, fusion, entry, to be infective
      - ❖ **Spike (gp120 glycoprotein) attache**s to CD4⁺ receptor on host cells (T cells, dendritic cells, macrophages); **gp41 transmembrane glycoprotein** facilitates fusion by attaching to a fusion receptor on the CD4⁺ cell
      - ❖ **Coreceptors** (CCR5 and CXCR4) needed
      - ❖ **Fusion:** the **gp41 transmembrane glycoprotein** participates in fusion of the **HIV** viral envelope with the cell
      - ❖ Entry pore made, following fusion
      - ❖ **Viral envelope** remains behind; **HIV uncoats** releasing **RNA core**
    - ✓ **Viral RNA** released and **transcribed into DNA** by **reverse transcriptase**
    - ✓ **Viral DNA** becomes **integrated** in the **host cells' chromosomal DNA**
    - ✓ **"DNA" can control production of new viruses or become a provirus**
    - ✓ **Provirus** may not be detected by the immune system; **may remain latent** (virus in vacuoles)
    - ✓ **Virus** undergoes antigenic changes to survive and have a high mutation rate
  - Clades (Subtypes) of **HIV**
    - ✓ **HIV-1:** currently three groups (based on viral genome) named: **M (main), O (outlier), N (non-M or non-O)**
      - ❖ **Group M:** cause of 95% global infections; thirteen (13) **clades**
    - ✓ **HIV-2:** mainly in western Africa
  - **The Stages of HIV Infection**
    - ✓ **AIDS:** the **final stage** of HIV infection
    - ✓ The progression of HIV divided into three phases
      - ❖ **Phase 1: HIV** population in blood rises; **billions of CD4+ T cells infected;** infection **asymptomatic or causes lymphadenopathy**
      - ❖ **Phase 2: CD4⁺ T cells decline; HIV replication continues; persistent infections** by *Candida albicans* (mouth, vagina, throat); shingles, persistent diarrhea, fever, **oral leukoplakia; cancers or precancerous lesions** of the cervix
      - ❖ **Phase 3: clinical AIDS emerges; CD4⁺ T cell counts below 350 cells/µl;** *Candida albicans* infecting esophagus, bronchi, lungs; CMV infecting eyes; *Pneumocystis* pneumonia; TB; Toxoplasmosis; Kaposi's sarcoma
    - ✓ **CDC** classifies progression **of HIV infections based on T cell populations**
      - ❖ Normal: 800 to 1000 CD4+ T cells/µl
      - ❖ **Below 350 cells/µl: indicating initial therapy with retroviral drugs**
      - ❖ **Below 200 cells/µl: diagnostic for AIDS**
      - ❖ **Progression** from initial HIV infection to AIDS **takes about ten (10) yrs**

- ■ **Resistance to HIV Infection**
  - ✓ **HIV** infection stimulates an initial strong and effective immune response: viral levels decline probably due to **CTLs (CD8⁺ T cells)**
- ■ **Survival with HIV Infection**
  - ✓ Infections by **opportunistic microbes**, due to an inadequate immune system, **leads to disease and death**
  - ✓ Success is treating the disease or condition; extends the lives of many HIV-infected persons
  - ✓ Older adults less able to replace **CD4+ T cell population;** infants and young children's immune system not fully developed
  - ✓ Infants born to HIV-positive mothers may not be infected
- ■ **Exposed, But Not Infected, Population**
  - ✓ Certain high risk individuals exposed to HIV, but remain infection free
  - ✓ 1% to 3% of the populations of the western world **do not have a gene for CCR5** (coreceptor used by HIV to enter and infect host cell), **therefore resistant to HIV infection**
  - ✓ Experiments underway to remove and modify some **T cells** by deleting **CCR5**
- ■ **Long-Term Survivors (Long-Term Nonprogressors)**
  - ✓ Certain therapeutically untreated individuals infected with HIV for greater than 10 years have not progressed to AIDS
  - ✓ Called **elite controllers**: have **CTLs** that are capable of destroying fast mutating viruses, like HIV

J. Diagnostic Methods
- ● **Standard procedure for detecting HIV antibodies: ELISA test** (most sensitive)
- ● **Positive screening test for antibodies then confirmed by Western blot test (HIV antigens by Western blotting)**
- ● Concern with testing is **seroconversion:** window of time between infection and detectable antibodies (about 21 to 25 days)
- ● Alternative to Western blot is **plasma viral load (PVL):** detects the **RNA of the HIV-1 virus** in blood; test can be used to also detect early HIV infections, before appearance of antibodies

K. HIV Transmission
- ● Requires **transfer of or direct contact with infected body fluids: blood and semen**
- ● Virus can survive 1.5 days inside a cell; 6 hours outside a cell
- ● Routes of transmission: sexual contact, transplacental to fetus, needles, breast milk, organ transplants, blood transfusions, artificial insemination
- ● **HIV** not transmitted by: insects, hugging, kissing, saliva, sharing household items

L. AIDS Worldwide
- ● **A global pandemic**
- ● Worldwide, **heterosexual transmission predominates; increasing percentage of women**
- ● Sub-Saharan Africa; South and Southeast Asia; China and India: Eastern Europe, Russia, and Central Asia; Western Europe and the United States
- ● North America, South America, Europe: transmission by male homosexual activity and injected drugs
- ● Eastern Europe, Central and Southeast Asia: transmission by injected drugs

M. The Prevention and Treatments of AIDS
- ● Practical means of control: **minimizing transmission**

- Through education; condoms; discouraging sexual promiscuity; sterile needles; medications
  - **HIV Vaccines: difficult**; virus remains viable inside host cells
  - **Chemotherapy:** progress made using chemotherapy in inhibit progression of infection
  - **Reverse transcriptase inhibitors:** [nucleoside reverse transcriptase inhibitors (**NRTIs**); **analogues of nucleosides;** cause termination of viral **DNA**]; [non-nucleoside reverse transcriptase inhibitors (**NNRTIs**); **not analogs of nucleosides**]
    - ✓ Current treatment termed: **highly active antiretroviral therapy (HAART)**: drug combinations
    - ✓ Examples: **Truvada** (tenofovir and emtricitabrine); **Atripla** (two drugs + efavirenz)
  - **Protease inhibitors: prevent proteases** from cleaving viral precursor proteins into smaller structural and functional proteins
    - ✓ Examples: **idinavir, atazanavir, saquinavir**
  - **Cell Entry Inhibitors:** drugs which prevent **attachment, fusion**
    - ✓ Examples: **enfuvirtide, maraviroc**
  - **Integrase Inhibitors:** inhibits **HIV integrase** (intergrates **cDNA** of HIV into host chromosome)
    - ✓ Example:**raltegravir**
  - **Maturation Inhibitors:** affects conversion of a precursor capsid to mature capsid
  - **Tetherins:** prevents release and spread of newly formed virus to the cell

N. The AIDS Epidemic and the Importance of Scientific Research
- Scientific research has been of great value in: identifying HIV as the causative agent of AIDS; developing tests for blood screening; understand and identify the viral life cycle; produce drugs for selective stages in the life cycle; monitor course of infection

MICROBIOLOGY

ANTIMICROBIAL DRUGS

A. The History of Chemotherapy
- **Antimicrobial drug:** any treatment which introduces a chemical substance into the body to destroy a pathogenic microbe, with minimal damage to host cells
- **Chemotherapy:** the treatment of disease by the use of chemical substances, especially the treatment of cancer by cytotoxic and other drugs
  - **Paul Ehrlich** developed concept of chemotherapy
- **Antibiotic:** a substance produced by microorganisms that inhibit another microorganism
  - **Alexander Fleming** discovered first antibiotic (**Penicillin)**
  - *Staphylococcus aureus* (bacterium) inhibited by *Penicillium notatum* (mold)
  - Representative sources of antibiotics: *Bacillus subtilis* (Bacitracin); *Streptomyces griseus* (Streptomycin); *Penicillium chrysogenum* (Penicillin)
- **Antibiotic Discovery Today**
  - Most antibiotics, were discovered by identifying and growing colonies of antibiotic-producing organisms, from soil samples

B. Spectrum of Antimicrobial Activity
- **Selective toxicity is important**
  - Find drugs that are **effective against prokaryotic cells; do not affect eukaryotic cells**
  - If the pathogen is an eukaryotic cell (fungus, protozoan, helminth), selective toxicity is more difficult
  - Viral infections difficult to treat
- **Narrow spectrum of microbial activity: Narrow range** of microbial types they affect
  - Example: **Penicillin G:** affects gram positive (+) bacteria, few gram negative (-) bacteria
- **Broad spectrum antibiotics: affects** a broad range of gram (+) bacteria or gram (-) bacteria
  - Example: **Tetracycline**
- **Superinfection:** can occur if pathogen becomes resistant to the drug, or when normally resistant microbiota multiply excessively
  - Example: overgrowth of *Candida albicans*

C. The Action of Microbial Drugs
- **Drugs either bactericidal** (kill microbe directly) **or bacteriostatic** (prevent microbes from growing)
  - **Inhibitors of Cell Wall Synthesis**
    - Inhibit the function and growth of the pathogens cell wall
    - Prevent the synthesis of peptidoglycan→weak cell wall→lyses
    - Affects only actively growing cells
    - **Penicillins**
      - ✓ Have a common core structure containing a **β-lactam ring,** but differ in their side chain; prevent cross linking of peptidoglycans
      - ✓ Can be produced **naturally or semisynthetically**
      - ✓ <u>Natural Penicillin</u>: extracted from cultures of mold *Penicillium*; **effective against gram positive (+) cocci and spirochetes**; disadvantages: narrow spectrum of activity and susceptible to **penicillinases** (β-lactamases)

- ❖ **Penicillin G:** prototype; narrow spectrum; when injected intramuscularly, rapidly excreted from the body in 3 to 6 hours
- ❖ **Procaine penicillin(Pen G + procaine):** retained up to 24 hours
- ❖ **Benzathine penicillin (Pen G + benzathine):** retained up to 4 months
- ❖ **Penicillin V:** stable in stomach acids; orally
  - ✓ **Semisynthetic Penicillin:** chemically altered natural Penicillins; broader spectrum of activity
    - ❖ **Penicillinase-Resistant Penicillins**
      *Methicillin: introduced; relatively resistant to the enzyme; resistance appeared; organisms eventually termed: methicillin-resistant *Staphylococcus aureus* **(MRSA)**
      *Oxacillin and Nafcillin: newer; to replace methicillin
    - ❖ **Extended-Spectrum Penicillins**
      *Ampicillin and Amoxicillin: broader spectrum (gram positive (+) and gram (-) negative); **not resistant to penicillinases**
      *Carbenicillin and Ticarcillin: broader spectrum against gram negative (-) and *Pseudomonas aeruginosa*
      *Mezlocillin and Azlocillin: modification of **ampicillin;** broader spectrum of activity
    - ❖ **Penicillins Plus β-Lactamase Inhibitors: combine penicillins with potassium clavulanate (clavulanic acid:** noncompetitive inhibitor of penicillinase; product of streptomycete)
      *Augmentin: combination of **amoxicillin** and **potassium clavulanate**
    - ❖ **Carbapenems:** substitute a carbon atom for a sulfur atom and add a double bond to the penicillin nucleus; broad spectrum of activity
      *Primaxin: combination to **imipenem** and **cilastin;** prevents breakdown by the kidneys
      *Doripenem: useful against *Pseudomonas aeruginosa*
    - ❖ **Monobactams:** has only a **single ring** rather than the B-lactam double ring
      *Aztreonam: low toxicity; affects only certain gram negative (-) bacteria: **including** *E. coli* and *Pseudomonads*
    - ❖ **Cephalosporins:** β-lactam ring differs from the penicillins; more widely used than any other β-lactam antibiotics
    - ❖ **Polypeptide Antibiotics**
      *Bacitracin: primarily effective against gram positive (+) bacteria; *Staphylococci* and *Streptococci*; **topical application**
      *Vancomycin: addresses **MRSA;** use has led to **vancomysin-resistant enterococci (VRE)**
- o **Antimycobacterial Antibiotics**
  - ■ Cell wall of genus *Mycobacterium* incorporates **mycolic acids** (stain Acid Fast positive)
    - ✓ **Isoniazid (INH):** effective against *Mycobacterium* tuberculosis; **inhibits synthesis of mycolic acid;** used in combination with other drugs to minimize resistance
    - ✓ **Rifampin:** used with **INH**
    - ✓ **Ethambutol:** used only against mycobacteria; inhibits incorporation of mycolic acid into the cell wall; **used as a secondary drug**
- o **Inhibitors of Protein Synthesis**
  - ■ Structure of ribosomes different: eukaryotic cells (80S) and **prokaryotic cells (70S)**
  - ■ Target the 70S ribosome made up of **a 50S and a 30S unit**
    - ✓ **Chloramphenicol**
      - ❖ Binds to **50S unit; inhibits peptide bond formation**

- ❖ Broad spectrum antibiotic
- ❖ Causes bone marrow suppression **(aplastic anemia)**
- ✓ **Clindamycin** and **metronidazole**: bind at same ribosomal site; inhibit protein synthesis
- ✓ **Aminoglycosides**: Interfere with the initial steps of protein synthesis; **change the shape of 30S unit** leading to incorrect coding on mRNA
  - ❖ Significant activity against **gram-negative (-) bacteria**
  - ❖ Disadvantage: **cause hearing and kidney damage**
  - ❖ **Streptomycin**: used to treat tuberculosis
  - ❖ **Neomycin: topical**
  - ❖ **Gentamicin**: *Pseudomonas aeruginosa*
  - ❖ **Tobramycin: aerosol;** aids patients with cystic fibrosis
- ✓ **Tetracyclines**: Broad spectrum antibiotic; **produced by** *Streptomyces* spp; interfere with the **attachment of tRNA carrying the amino acids to the ribosome at the 30S unit**
  - ❖ UTI's, rickettsial infections, chlamydia infections, mycoplasma pneumonia; alternate drug for syphilis and gonorrhea
  - ❖ Added to animal feeds
  - ❖ Disadvantage: **teeth discoloration; liver damage**
  - ❖ **Oxytetracycline** (Terramycin)
  - ❖ **Chlortetracycline** (Aueromycin)
  - ❖ **Tetracycline**
  - ❖ **Doxycycline** and **Minocycline**: semisynthetic tetracyclines
- ✓ **Glycylcyclines**: structurally similar to tetracyclines; newly discovered
  - ❖ **Tygecycline** (Tygacil); broad-spectrum; **bacteriostatic; binds to 30S unit;** administered by slow intravenous infusion; useful against **MRSA** and *Actinetobacter baumanii*
- ✓ **Macrolides**: have a **macrocyclic lactone ring**
  - ❖ **Erythromycin**: best known; **alternative to penicillin;** can be administered orally; drug of choice to treat legionellosis, mycoplasmal pneumonia; streptococcal and staphylococcal infection in children
  - ❖ **Azithromycin and Clarithromycin**: broader antimicrobial spectrum; *Chlamydia*
- ✓ **Streptogramins: new;** developed to combat vancomycin resistant pathogens
  - ❖ **Synercid:** combination of quinupristin and dalfopristin (both cyclic peptides) which block protein synthesis by attaching to the **50S unit,** but at different points; effective against a broad range of **gram positive (+) bacteria that are resistant to other antibiotics**
- ✓ **Oxazolidinones: new;** developed in response to vancomycin resistance; act on the ribosome; synthetic
  - ❖ **Linezolid** (Zyvox): **new;** used for **MRSA**
- ✓ **Pleuromutilins: new**
  - ❖ **Mutilin and Retpamulin**: both target same point on the ribosome as the macrolides; effective against **gram positive (+) bacteria**

- o **Injury to the Plasma Membrane**
  - ■ Brings changes in the **permeability** of the plasma membrane, leading to **loss of metabolites** important to the microbial cell
  - ■ Synthesis of plasma membrane requires the synthesis of fatty acids as building blocks; several antibiotic are focused on this process
    - ✓ **Isoniazid (INH)** and **Triclosan**: successful antimicrobials which target fatty acid synthesis
    - ✓ **Lipopeptides: new** class of antibiotics

❖ **Daptomycin:** antibiotic; active against **gram positive (+) bacteria;** attacks membrane resulting in structural changes, leading to arrest of synthesis of DNA, RNA, proteins; **MRSA**
✓ **Polymyxin B:** effective against **gram negative (-) bacteria;** *Pseudomonas*: used **topically**
✓ **Polymyxin B** and **Bacitracin:** both available in nonprescription antiseptic ointments; usually combined with **neomycin**

o **Inhibitors of Nucleic Acid Synthesis**
  ■ **Interfere with DNA/RNA replication and transcription**
    ✓ **Rifamycins (Rifampin):inhibit synthesis of mRNA;** reach the CSF; treat tuberculosis and leprosy; side effects: feces, urine, sweat, saliva, tears turn orange-red
    ✓ **Quinolones and Fluoroguinolones**
      ❖ **Nalidixic acid:** first of the quinolone group; interferes with **DNA gyrase** (needed for replication of DNA): limited use to treats UTI's
      ❖ **Fluoroquinolones:** synthetic quinolones; divided into two groups, each with a broader spectrum of activity; relatively nontoxic
        *Norfloxacin and Ciprofloxacin (Cipro): Cipro used against anthrax infections
        *Gatifloxacin, Gemifloxacin, and Moxifloxacin: for UTI's and certain pneumonias (except Moxifloxacin)
o **Competitive Inhibitors of the Synthesis of Essential Metabolites**
  ■ **Compete using a substance (antimetabolite) which resembles the normal substrate**
    ✓ **Sulfonamides** (or sulfa drugs); usually bacteriostatic; structure similar to **para-amino benzoic acid (PABA);** continue to be used to treat **certain UTI's;** used in the **combination** with **drug silver sulfadiazine,** which is **used to control infections in burn victims;**
    ✓ **Trimethoprim** and **Sulfamethoxazole (TMP-SMZ):** used for **gram negative (-) pathogens for UTI's and intestinal tract infections;** example of drug **synergism**
o **Antifungal Drugs**
  ■ Fungi are eukaryotic; use same mechanisms to synthesize proteins and nucleic acids
  ■ **Agents affecting Fungal Sterols:** target **sterols** (in fungi, mainly **ergosterol**) in plasma membrane
    ✓ **Polyenes:** target ergosterol in the plasma membrane→ permeability→ death
      ❖ **Amphotericin B:** produced by *Streptomyces* species; for systemic diseases such as histoplasmosis, blastomycosis, coccidioidomycosis; **toxic to kidneys;** administered in liposomes to decrease toxicity
    ✓ **Azoles:** interfere with ergosterol synthesis
      ❖ **Imidazoles**
        *Clotrimazole and Miconazole: topical use for cutaneous mycoses, vaginal yeast infections
        *Ketoconazole: broad spectrum of activity among fungi; topical use (dermatomycosis of the skin); orally for systemic infections; liver damage
        *Triazole, Fluconazole, and Itraconazole: less toxic than Ketoconazole
        *Voriconazole: primarily *Aspergillus*
        *Posaconazole: newest
      ❖ **Allylamines:** unique way inhibiting biosynthesis of **ergosterols**
        *Terbinafine and naftifine: used when resistance to azole-type antifungals arises
  ■ **Agents affecting Fungal Cell Walls**
    ✓ **Echinocandins:** attacks β-**glucan** (component of the **cell wall**) →incomplete cell wall→ lyses
      ❖ **Caspofungin (Cancidas):** systemic *Aspergillus*, *Candida* spp

- **Agents inhibiting Nucleic Acids**
  - ✓ **Flucytosine:** interferes with biosynthesis of **RNA**; fungal cell converts **flucytosine** into **5-fluoruracil**→ disrupts proteins synthesis; toxic to kidneys and bone marrow
- **Other Antifungal Drugs**
  - ✓ **Griseofulvin: blocks microtubule assembly;** produced by species of *Penicillium*; used for superficial dermatophytic fungal infections (tinea capitis, nails); given **orally**
  - ✓ **Tonaftate:** alternative **to miconazole**; athlete's foot; mechanism unknown
  - ✓ **Undecylenic acid:** fatty acid with antifungal activity
  - ✓ **Pentamidine:** appears to bind to DNA; treatment of *Pneumocystis* pneumonia and several protozoan-caused tropical diseases

- o **Antiviral Drugs**
  - Difficult to target the virus without harming/damaging the host's own cells
  - Many antiviral drugs directed against HIV
  - Many antivirals used today are **analogs** of components of **viral DNA or RNA**
  - **Nucleoside and Nucleotide Analogs**
    - ✓ **Interfere** with the **synthesis of viral DNA or RNA**
      - ❖ **Acyclovir** (nucleoside analog): treats genital herpes
      - ❖ **Famciclovir** (taken orally) and **Ganciclovir:** derivatives of Acyclovir
      - ❖ **Ribavirin:** resembles nucleoside **guanine;** accelerates the mutation rate of **RNA viruses**
      - ❖ **Lamivudine** (nucleoside): treats Hepatitis B
      - ❖ **Adefovir dipivoxil (Hepsera): nucleotide analog**
      - ❖ **Ganciclovir** (nucleoside analog): used to treat CMV
      - ❖ **Cidofovir:** (nucleoside analog): **currently used to treat CMV infections;** possibly **smallpox**
  - **Other Enzyme Inhibitors**
    - ✓ **Inhibit the enzyme neuraminidase**
      - ❖ **Zanamivir (Relenza)** and **Oseltamivir (Tamiflu):** treatment for influenza
  - **Antivirals for Treating HIV/AIDS**
    - ✓ Targeted at the enzyme **reverse transcriptase,** which controls the synthesis of RNA from DNA
    - ✓ **Antiretroviral:** drug used to treat HIV infections
      - ❖ **Zidovudine** (nucleoside analog): for HIV infection
      - ❖ **Tenofovir** (nucleotide analog): **only nucleotide reverse transcriptase inhibitor**
      - ❖ **Atripla:** combines **Tenofovir, Emtricitabine,** and **Efavirenz**
      - ❖ **Nevirapine:** non-nucleoside agent; **blocks RNA synthesis** via other mechanisms
    - ✓ **Protease Inhibitors:** competitively inhibit **proteases** from cutting up large proteins into fragments used to assemble new viruses
      - ❖ **Atazanavir, Indinavir, Saquinavir:** effective when **combined with inhibitors** or **reverse transcriptase**
    - ✓ **Integrase Inhibitors:** inhibit an enzyme that intergrates viral DNA into the DNA of the infected cell
      - ❖ **Raltegravir**
    - ✓ **Entry Inhibitors:** targets the **receptors** which HIV binds to cell **before entry (CCR5)**
      - ❖ **Maraviroc**
    - ✓ **Fusion Inhibitors:** blocks entry of HIV into the cell
      - ❖ **Enfuvirtide:** mimics region of the **gp41 HIV-1 envelope**
  - **Interferons**
    - ✓ Produced by cells infected by a virus; inhibit further spread of the infection

        ✓ **Interferons** classified as **cytokines**
        ❖ **Alpha interferon:** used to treat **viral Hepatitis**
      ✓ **Imiquimod:** antiviral drug; stimulates production of interferon; used to treat **genital warts**

- o **Antiprotozoan and Antihelminth Drugs**
  - ■ **Antiprotozoan Drugs**
    - ✓ **Quinine:** still used to treat malaria
    - ✓ **Chloroquine: synthetic** replacement for quinine
    - ✓ **Mefloquine (Lariam):** used when there is resistance to chloroquine
    - ✓ **Artemisinin** and **Artemisinin-based** combination therapies **(ACTs):** principle treatment of malaria; expensive
    - ✓ **Quinacrine:** drug of choice to treat **giardiasis**
    - ✓ **Diiodohydroxyquin (Iodoquinol):** intestinal amoebic diseases; damages optic nerve
    - ✓ **Metronidazole (Flagyl):** used against parasitic **protozoans** (*Trichomonas vaginalis*, giardiasis, amoebic dysentery) **and obligate anaerobic bacteria** (*Clostridium*)
    - ✓ **Tinidazole:** similar to **metronidazole**; treats giardiasis, amoebiasis, and trichomoniasis
    - ✓ **Nitazoxanide:** used to treat diarrhea caused by *Crytosporidium homonis*; giardiasis and amoebiasis; several **helminthic diseases**; some anaerobic bacteria
  - ■ **Antihelminthic Drugs**
    - ✓ **Niclosamide:** first choice in treatment of **tapeworms; inhibits ATP** production under aerobic conditions
    - ✓ **Praziquantel:** treatment of **tapeworms; alters permeability** of the plasma membrane; causes helminthes to undergo **muscular spasms** and make them **susceptible to host immune system;** used to treat fluke-caused diseases, especially schistosomiasis
    - ✓ **Mebendazole and Albendazole:** inhibit **microtubule formation;** used to treat intestinal helminthic infections; widely used in livestock industry
    - ✓ **Ivermectin:** produced by *Streptomyces avermectinius*; effective against many **nematodes** (roundworms), **several mites** (such as scabies), **ticks, head lice;** causes **paralysis and death** of the **helminth**

D. Tests to Guide Chemotherapy

- ● Susceptibility of pathogenic microbes can change over time (resistance)
- ● Several tests are used to determine which chemotherapeutic drug combats a particular pathogen
- ● These tests help determine which antibiotic is to be prescribed
  - o **Diffusion Methods**
    - ■ One places a paper disc or plastic strip that is coated with a chemotherapeutic agent in touch with a pathogen to determine if the agent inhibits the pathogen
    - ■ **Disk-diffusion method** (Kirby-Bauer test)
      - ✓ **Disks** impregnated with the **chemotherapeutic agent; placed in petri dish** evenly seeded with a test organism
      - ✓ Dish incubated; chemotherapeutic agent diffuses from **disks**
      - ✓ If **agent effective, zone of inhibition** (clear zone) **seen** and diameter measured
      - ✓ Diameter of zone measured and compared to a standard table
      - ✓ Standard table indicates whether pathogen is: sensitive, intermediate, or resistant to the agent
      - ✓ Test is simple and inexpensive; results often inadequate
    - ■ **E Test**
    - ■ More advanced diffusion method
    - ■ Allows one to estimate the **minimal inhibitory concentration (MIC):** determines the **lowest concentration of the chemotherapeutic agent which inhibits visible growth**

- A plastic **coated strip** (contains an increasing gradient of the chemotherapeutic agent) placed on an agar surface, seeded with the test organism
- **MIC** can be read
  - o **Broth Dilution Methods**
    - Determine the **MIC** and the **minimal bactericidal concentration (MBC)** of the chemotherapeutic agent
    - **MBC: the lowest concentration** of a chemotherapeutic agent needed **to kill a pathogen**
      - ✓ **MIC** determined by making a **sequence of decreasing concentrations of the drug** in a broth which is then inoculated with the pathogen, and incubated
      - ✓ Wells showing no growth (**higher concentration** than the **MIC**) can be cultured in broth or agar plates free of drug
      - ✓ If **growth occurs, drug not bacteriocidal,** and the **MBC** can be determined
      - ✓ **MIC and MBC** avoid misuse of expensive antibiotics and minimize chance of toxicity
  - o **Antibiograms:** periodic reports which record susceptibility of organisms encountered clinically

E. Resistance to Antimicrobial Drugs

- First exposure to a new antibiotic causes the susceptibility and mortality rate of microbes to be very high, leaving a few survivors
- This survival usually due to genetic changes, which allows **progeny to become resistant**
- This genetic change arises from **random mutations**
- **Drug resistance** often carried by **plasmids, or transposons**
- Bacteria resistant to large number of antibiotics called **superbugs** (Examples: **MRSA**, *Enterococcus faecium, Staphylococcus aureus, Pseudomonas aeruginosa*)
- **Mechanisms of Resistance**
  - o **Enzymatic Destruction or Inactivation of the drug:** mainly affects antibiotics that are natural products
    - Examples: penicillin, cephalosporins, cabapenans; all share the β-**lactam ring** which is the target for β-**lactamase** (enzyme produced by bacteria)
    - **Penicillinase-resistant** drugs later produced (Example: methicillin, vancomycin)
    - **MRSA** (outbreaks in the community) produce a toxin (**leukocidin**) which destroys neutrophils
  - o **Prevention of Penetration to Target Site within the Microbe**
    - Because of makeup of **cell wall (gram negative (-)** bacteria), can't be penetrated; some bacterial **mutants modify porins** making entrance by antibiotics impossible
  - o **Target Site Within Microbe Altered**
    - Minor modifications affecting protein synthesis at, certain sites can **neutralize** effects of antibiotics
    - **MRSA:** gained resistance by modifying the **penicillin-binding protein (PBP);** B-lactam antibiotics acted by binding with the PBP
  - o **Rapid Efflux (Ejection) of the Antibiotic**
    - **Gram negative (-) bacteria** contain certain proteins which act as **pumps,** in the plasma membrane; **expels** antibiotics
  - o **Variations of Mechanisms of Resistance**
    - A microbe can become resistant by synthesizing large amounts of the enzyme against which the drug is targeted (Example: resistance to trimethoprim)
    - A microbe can become resistant by producing smaller amounts of sterols against the drug which is effective (Example: polyene antibiotics)
- **Antibiotic Misuse**
  - o Antibiotics are misused; prescribed for the wrong reason (for headaches)
  - o Not necessarily prescribed by the correct medical provider

- o Certain medications can be purchased without a prescription
- o Dosages given incorrectly and/or taken incorrectly
- o Not to treat disease, but used in animal feeds to promote growth
- **Cost and Prevention of Resistance**
  - o Antibiotic resistance is costly
  - o Developing newer drugs costly
  - o Stratergies to prevent development of resistance: **finish full regimen of prescription; never use relic antibiotics to treat a new illness; ensure choice and dose are appropriate; prescribe most specific antibiotic possible; hospitals, nursing homes, clinics have special monitoring committees to review the use, effectiveness, and cost of antibiotics**

F. Antibiotic Safety

- One must consider the risks of the **"side effects" versus "benefits"**
- Side effects may be serious involving **liver, kidney, hearing, teeth**
- The **Therapeutic index:** an assessment of risks against benefits when administering a drug
  - o Examples: pregnancy; hypersensitivity reactions (penicillin); drug taken alone or in combination

G. Effects of Combinations of Drugs

- The effects of two or more drugs given simultaneously is sometimes greater than the effect of either drug given alone; this effect called **synergism**
  - o Example: penicillin and streptomycin for bacterial endocarditis
- Other combination of some drugs can show less effectiveness ; effect called **antagonism**
  - o Example: penicillin and tetracycline; better effectiveness when used alone

H. The Future of Chemotherapeutic Agents

- Microbes are becoming resistant
- Drugs need to be modified to extend their spectrum
- Identifying different targets for antimicrobial action
- Much research now looking at microbial genome
- Focusing on the production of antibiotics using plants, mammals, birds, amphibians, to produce a new class of **antimicrobial peptides**
  - o **Antimicrobial peptides:** part of defense systems of most forms of life
    - Amphibians: **magainins:** attacks bacterial membranes
    - Sharks: **squalamine:** antimicrobial substance
- Phage Therapy: certain **bacteriophage** capable of killing certain bacteria

MICROBIOLOGY

MICROBIAL DISEASES OF THE SKIN AND EYES

A. Structure and Function of the Skin
- Covers and protects body
- First defense against pathogen
- Consist of **two principle parts**
  - **Epidermis:** effective physical **barrier against microbes**
    - Thin outer portion: layers of epithelial cells
    - Outermost layer of **epidermis** called **stratum corneum:** consists of dead cells containing **keratin**
  - **Dermis:** composed **mostly of connective tissue**
    - Inner thick layer
    - Hair follicles, oil glands, sweat ducts located (passageways in which microbes can enter)
- Perspiration: provides moisture and nutrients for some microbial growth; also contains salts, lysozymes, and antimicrobial peptides, all which inhibit many microbes
- Sebum: mixture of lipids, proteins, and salts which prevent skin and hair from drying out; also a nutritive for certain microbes

B. Mucous Membranes
- **Lines body cavities** (GI, respiratory, urinary, genital)
- Differs from skin: consists of sheets of **tightly packed epithelial cells** attached at their bases to a layer of extracellular material called a **basement membrane**
- Many of these cells secrete **mucus (**hence the name **mucous membrane or mucosa)**
- Some **mucosal cells** have cilia (traps and sweep microbes and particles out of body)
- Often acidic, limiting microbial growth
- Membranes of the eyes washed by tears (tears contain lysozyme) which limit microbial growth

C. Normal Microbiota of the Skin
- Supports the growth of certain microbes
- Consist of large numbers of **gram positive (+) bacteria: staphylococci and micrococci**
  - **Gram positive (+) cocci** relatively resistant to drying and high osmotic pressures
- Consist of **gram positive (+) pleomorphic rods** called **diphtheroids**
  - *Propionibacterium acnes*: **anaerobic**; inhabit hair follicles
  - *Corynebacterium xerosis*: **aerobic**; occupy skin surface
- Few **gram negative (-) bacteria**
  - *Acinetobacter*: colonizes the skin
- **Yeast**
  - *Malassezia furfur*: grows on oily skin secretions; thought to be the cause of **dandruff**

D. Microbial Diseases of the Skin
- **Lesions** described as:
  - **Vesicles:** small, fluid-filled
  - **Bullae:** vesicles larger than 1 cm in diameter
  - **Macules:** flat, reddened lesions

- o **Papules:** raised lesions
- o **Pustules:** contain pus
- **Rashes** described as:
- o **Exanthem: skin** rash arising from disease conditions
- o **Enanthem:** rash on **mucosal surface (mucosa)**
- **Bacterial Diseases of the Skin**
- o **Staphylococcal Skin Infections**
    - Gram positive (+) round or spherical bacteria in clusters like grapes
    - Divided into two groups depending on their ability to produce **coagulase** (enzyme that clots fibrin in blood) or not
        - ✓ **Coagulase Negative Strains**
            - ❖ *Staphylococcus epidermidis:* common on skin (90% of normal microbiota); infection caused by broken skin due to insertion or removal of **catheters into veins**
        - ✓ **Coagulase Positive Strains**
            - ❖ *Staphylococcus aureus:* most pathogenic; permanent resident of nasal passages of 20% of the population; forms yellow-golden colonies; able to form **coagulase, damaging toxins;** some strains cause **sepsis;** others produce **enterotoxins;** some infections include:

            ***Folliculitis:** enters body through hair follicle

            ***Sty:** infected follicle of eyelash

            ***Furuncle (boil):** type of **abscess** (localized region of pus surrounded by inflamed tissue)

            ***Carbuncle:** extensive **furuncle;** hard, deep round inflammation of tissue under the skin

            ***Impetigo:** highly contagious; affects children 2 to 5 years of age; two forms
            - ➢ Nonbullous impetigo: isolated pustules which become crusted
            - ➢ Bullous impetigo: caused by staphylococcal toxin; a localized form of **scalded skin syndrome** (caused by exfoliative toxin); in hospital nurseries, known as **pemphigus neonatorum**

            ***Toxic shock syndrome:** fever, vomiting, sunburn-like rash, followed by shock and sometimes organ failure; **toxic shock syndrome toxin 1 (TSST-1)** is formed; associated with **tampons and nasal absorbent packing**
- o **Streptococcal Skin Infections**
    - Gram positive (+) round or spherical bacteria usually grows in chains
    - Secrete **toxins (hemolysins)** and **enzymes**
    - **Hemolysin:** lyses not only red blood cells, but any type of cell
    - Depending on **hemolysin** they produce, streptococcus categorized as **alpha (α), beta (β), or gamma (γ)/nonhemolytic**
        - ✓ **β-Hemolytic Streptococci**
            - ❖ Associated with human disease
            - ❖ Further differentiated, **A through T**, according to antigenic carbohydrates in cell wall
            - ❖ **Group A streptococci (GAS):** synonymous with species *Streptococcus pyogenes;* most common human pathogen; divided into immunological types according to antigenic properties of the **M protein;** capsule of hyaluronic acid; produce **streptokinases, hyaluronidase, deoxyribonucleases, steptolysins;** some infections include:

            ***Erysipelas:** infects dermal layer; skin erupts into red patches with raised margins; can progress to sepsis; sensitive to cephalosporins

> > > ***Necrotizing fasciitis:** extensive destruction of the fascia; systemic toxicity; **exotoxin A** (acts as a superantigen)
> > > ***Streptococcal toxic shock syndrome (streptococcal TSS):** associated with necrotizing fasciitis; bacteremia; damaging enzymes released leading to shock and organ damage; mortality rate higher than staphylococcal TTS
> > > ***Impetigo:** caused by **GAS**

- o **Infections by Pseudomonads**
    - Pseudomonads are aerobic gram negative (-) rods; in soil and water; resistant to many antibiotics and disinfectants; can grow on soap films
        - ✓ *Pseudomonas aeruginosa:* most prominent species; opportunistic pathogen; produce several **exotoxins**; has an **endotoxin;** grows in a **biofilm;** opportunistic pathogen for cystic fibrosis patients, burn patients; blue green pus (due to **pyocyanin**); treated with: quinolones, anti-pseudomonal β-lactam antibiotics, silver sulfadiazine; infections include:
            - ❖ **Pseudomonas dermatitis:** self-limiting rash (last about two weeks); associated with swimming pools, pool-type saunas, hot tubes
            - ❖ **Otitis externa:** or swimmer's ear
- o **Buruli Ulcer**
    - Caused by *Mycobacterium ulcerans:* similar to mycobacteria that causes tuberculosis and leprosy; disease progresses slowly with few side effects; leads to deep ulcer with extensive tissue damage due to **toxin, mycolactone**; associated with: swamps, slow-flowing waters; diseases include:
        - ✓ **Buruli ulcer:** primarily in western and central Africa; Mexico and areas of South America
- o **Acne**
    - *Propionibacterium acnes:* an anaerobic diphtheroid; commonly found on skin
    - Most common skin disease in humans; primarily teenagers
    - Develops when cells inside hair follicle shed at a higher number, than normal; combine with sebum causing follicles to clog
    - Causes include: increase cell turnover, sebum accumulation, bacteria, hormones
    - Classification: **comedonal (mild) acne, Inflammatory (moderate) acne, Nodular cystic (severe) acne**
        - ✓ **Comedonal (mild):** treated with: topical agents, Clear Light, Laser Systems; agents do not interfere with sebum formation
        - ✓ **Inflammatory (moderate):** arises from bacterial action; bacteria metabolize **glycerol in sebum;** leads to free fatty acids causing inflammation; inflammation produces pustules and papules; therapy at preventing sebum production and targeting bacteria (benzoyl peroxide, clindamycin (BenzaClin), erythromycin (Benzamycin), and Epiduo (Adapalene and benzoyl peroxide), Clear Light and Laser Systems
        - ✓ **Nodular Cystic (severe):** nodules or cyst filled with inflamed pus; leaves scars; effective treatment: **isotretinoin (Accutane),** but highly teratogenic
- ● **Viral diseases of the Skin**
    - o **Papillomavirus:** 50 types; causes several types of **warts** (or called **papillomas**); generally benign; transmitted by contact, even sexually; treatments: cryotherapy, electrodessication, burn with acids, podofilox, imiquimod (Aldara), lasers, bleomycin; associated with some skin and cervical cancers
    - o **Smallpox (Variola) Virus:** two forms (**variola major** and **variola minor**); transmitted via respiratory route; eradicated due to worldwide vaccination (WHO); concern as an agent for bioterrorism; complications from vaccine treated with vaccinia immune globulin or cidofovir

- o **Monkeypox:** similar to **smallpox** in symptoms; known to jump from animals to humans; human to human transmission very limited; occasional outbreaks; vaccination for smallpox protects
- o **Chickenpox (Varicella) and Shingles (Herpes Zoster)**
  - **Chickenpox (Varicella):** childhood disease; result from initial infection with **herpesvirus varicella-zoster(human herpesvirus 3)**; enters via respiratory system, then to localized skin cells; initially a vesicle→eventually forms a scab, then heals; complications: pneumonia or encephalitis, if pregnant fetal damage
    - ✓ **Reye's syndrome:** severe complication; persistent vomiting, brain dysfunction, coma and death; associated with the use of aspirin to lower fever
- o **Chickenpox (Varicella) and Shingles (Herpes Zoster) (Cont.)**
  - **Shingles (Herpes Zoster):** different expression of the virus; virus can remain latent (enters peripheral nerves, moves to central ganglion remaining dormant); can be reactivated; move to cutaneous sensory nerves causing outbreak in the form of **shingles (Herpes Zoster)**; vesicles localized in distinctive areas (**dermatomes**); can result into **postherpetic neuralgia**; antiviral drugs used: acyclovir, valacyclovir, and famciclovir; partially effective live, attenuated vaccine used
- o **Herpes Simplex Virus (HSV):** two groups **HSV-1(humans herpesvirus 1)** and **HSV-2 (human herpesvirus 2)**
  - **HSV-1 (or human herpesvirus-1):** transmitted orally or by respiratory route; remains dormant in the trigeminal nerve ganglia; develop lesions known as cold sores or fever blisters; triggered by UV radiation from sun, emotional stress, hormonal changes; associated with **herpes gladiatorum** and **herpetic whitlow**
  - **HSV-2 (or humans herpesvirus-2):** transmitted by sexual contact; causes genital herpes; latent in the sacral nerve
  - **HSV-1 and HSV-2:** can cause **herpes encephalitis**
- o **Measles (Rubeola):** extremely contagious; almost eliminated due to vaccine (**MMR**); symptoms resemble common cold; macular rash appears (begins on face→spreading to trunk and extremities); **Koplik's spots** (red spots with central blue-white specks on oral mucosa); complications include: middle ear infections, pneumonia, encephalitis; **subacute sclerosing panencephalitis**
- o **German measles (Rubella):** milder than measles; transmitted by respiratory route; macular rash of small red spots and fever; complications: **congenital rubella syndrome** (maternal infection during first trimester), encephalitis (rare); vaccine introduced since 1969 (not for pregnant women)
- o **Other Viral Rashes**
  - **Fifth Disease (Erythema Infectiosum):** caused by **human parvirus B19;** produces **"slapped cheek"** facial rash which slowly fades; can cause anemia, episodic arthritis, or miscarriage, in adults
  - **Roseola Roseola:** caused by **human herpesviruses 6 (HHV-6) and human herpesvirus 7 (HHV-7);** both viruses present in saliva of most adults; common in children; fever followed by rash over most of body lasting 1 or 2 days
- ● **Fungal diseases of the Skin and Nails**
  - o **Mycosis:** any fungal infection of the body
  - o **Cutaneous Mycoses**
    - **Dermatophytes:** fungi colonizing hair, nails, and stratum corneum; grow on keratin
    - **Dermatomycoses: cause fungal infections**
      - ✓ **Tinea capitis:** ringworm of scalp; can lead to baldness
      - ✓ **Tinea cruris:** ringworm of the groin or jock itch
      - ✓ **Tinea pedis:** ringworm of the foot or athlete's foot
      - ✓ **Tinea unguium (onychomycosis):** ringworm of the nail bed

- Three genera involved in cutaneous mycosis
  - ❖ *Trichophyton*: infect hair, skin, or nails
  - ❖ *Microsporum*: usually only hair or skin
  - ❖ *Epidermophyton*: only skin and nails
- Topical treatments: miconazole, clotrimazole; allylamine preparations containing terbinafine, naftifine, or butenavine; griseofulvin (oral); oral itraconazole and terbinafine for tinea unguium

  o **Subcutaneous Mycoses**
  - Usually from fungi **living in soil**; penetrate the skin thru small wound
  - *Sporothrix schenkii*: causes **sporotrichosis;** a dimorphic fungus; occurs among gardeners or those working with soil; spread to lymphatics; produce subcutaneous nodules; treated by ingesting dilute solution of potassium iodide

  o **Candidiasis**
  - Such fungi as *Candida albicans* growth usually suppressed by normal microbiota of mucous membranes of the GU tract and mouth; overgrowth can be due to: antibiotic use; change in mucosal pH; immunosuppressed individuals (AIDS); obese or diabetic persons
  - *Candida tropicalis* or *Candida krusei* : may also be involved
  - **Candidiasis:** overgrowth by *Candida albicans*
  - **Thrush:** white overgrowth of the oral cavity, seen in newborn infants
  - **Vaginitis:** common cause of infection by *Candida albicans*
  - Treatment: topical miconazole, clotrimazole, nystatin; fluconazole (system disease); new drugs include: micafungin, anidulafungin

- **Parasitic infestation of the Skin**
  o Includes protozoa, helminths, arthropods (microscopic)
  - **Scabies:** caused by **the mite** *Sarcoptes scabiei*; burrows under skin to lay eggs; transmitted by intimate contact (sexual, nursing home residents, baby sitters**); causes intense itching; treated with: permethin or oral ivermectin
  - **Pediculosis:** caused by **lice;** *Pediculus humanus capitus* (head lice), *Pediculus humanus corporis* (body lice); lice require blood; causes itching; eggs attached to hair shafts, vary in stages; treatment: combing; Nix (permethin) and Rid (pyrethrin): both insecticides; malathion (Ovide); lindane (toxic); ivermectin; dimethicone

E. Microbial diseases of the Eye
- Many microbes infect the eye mainly through the **conjunctiva** (mucous membrane)
  o **Inflammation of the Eye Membrane: Conjunctivitis**
  - **Conjunctivitis (Red eye or Pink eye):** inflammation of the conjunctiva
  - *Haemophilus influenza*: most common bacterial cause
  - Adenoviruses: viral cause
  - Pseudomonads: infections associated with contact lens

  o **Bacterial Diseases of the Eye**
  - **Opthalmia Neonatorum:** caused by *Neisseria gonorrhoeae*; spread via enfant passing through birth canal; can lead to ulceration of the cornea; blindness; treatment: antibiotics, povidone-iodine dilute solution
  - **Inclusion conjunctivitis:** caused by *Chlamydia trachomatis* (obligate intracellular parasite); infants exposed through birth canal; can cause blindness; can spread thru unchlorinated waters in swimming pools; treated with tetracycline ointment
  - **Trachoma:** caused by certain serotypes of *Chlamydia trachomatis*: can lead to blindness; spread by hand contact or sharing personal objects; flies may be carriers; can lead to **trichiasis** (in-turning of eyelashes); treatment: oral azithromycin

- o **Herpetic keratitis**
    - ■ Caused by **Herpes Simplex Type 1 virus (HSV-1)**; can infect the **cornea;** resulting in ulcers; blindness; treatment: trifluridine
- o **Acanthamoeba keratitis**
    - ■ Found in fresh and tap water, hot tubes, soil; associated with contact lenses; causes inflammation of the **cornea;** could lead to damage; treatment: propamidine isethionate eyedrops, topical neomycin; corneal transplant or eye removal

MICROBIOLOGY

MICROBIAL DISEASES OF THE CENTRAL NERVOUS SYSTEM

A. Structure and Function of the Nervous System
- Control center of the entire body
  - **Central Nervous System (CNS):** brain and spinal cord
  - **Peripheral Nervous System (PNS):** nerves branching off the brain and spinal cord
  - **Meninges:** covers and protects brain and spinal cord; consist of
    - Dura mater
    - Arachnoid mater
      - ✓ Subarachnoid space: CSF
    - Pia mater
  - **Blood brain barrier:** capillaries permitting certain substances to pass from the blood into the brain
  - **Meningitis:** inflammation of the meninges
  - **Encephalitis:** inflammation of the brain
  - **Meningoencephalitis:** inflammation of the brain and meninges

B. Bacterial Diseases of the Nervous System
- **Bacterial Meningitis**
  - Symptoms: fever, headache, stiff neck, nausea/vomiting; can lead to convulsions and coma
    - **Haemophilus influenza Meningitis**
      - ✓ *Haemophilus influenza*: aerobic; gram negative (-); carbohydrate capsule; normal throat microbiota; enters blood stream; children (6 months to 4 years of age)
    - **Neisseria Meningitis (Meningococcal Meningitis)**
      - ✓ *Neisseria meningitides*: aerobic gram negative (-); polysaccharide capsule; present in nose and throat ; throat infection leading to bacteremia; occurs in: children under 2 years of age, college students, dormitories, barracks; six capsular serotypes associated with disease are (A, B, C, W-135, X, Y); treatment: vaccines (except for serotype B)
    - **Streptococcal Meningitis (Pneumococcal Meningitis)**
      - ✓ *Streptococcus pneumoniae*: gram positive (+); encapsulated diplococcus; common in children 1 month to 4 years old; treatment: conjugated vaccine
    - **Diagnosis and Treatment of Most Common Types of Bacterial Meningitis**
      - ✓ Sample from **CSF**; Gram stain
      - ✓ Broad spectrum third-generation cephalosporins first choice; vancomycin
    - **Listeriosis**
      - ✓ *Listeria monocytogenes*: gram positive (+) rod; cause stillbirths, neurological disease in animals; in soil and water via animal feces; 4th most common cause of bacterial meningitis; affects fetus, newborn, adult; can cause sepsis; outbreaks in humans (foodborne ready to eat deli meats, dairy products) grows at refrigeration temperatures; treatment: Penicillin G
- **Tetanus**
  - *Clostridium tetani*: gram positive (+) rod; obligate anaerobic; endospore; common in soil contaminated with animal feces; symptoms caused by **tetanospasmin** (neurotoxin) which blocks relaxation pathway causing **muscle spasms** (Examples: **lockjaw, opisthotonos**); treatment: vaccination (a toxoid), tetanus immune globulin (TIG), debridement

- **Botulism**
  - *Clostridium botulinum*: gram positive (+) rod; obligate anaerobic; endospore; found in soil, aquatic sediments; anaerobic environment (sealed food cans) produces endospores which produce an **exotoxin**(neurotoxin: specific for the synaptic end of the nerve) which blocks releases of acetylcholine (a neurotransmitter); causes: double vision, difficulty swallowing, **flaccid paralysis**; a form of food poisoning; treatment: boiling food, nitrates (preservative) added, acidic environments
    - **Serological Types of Botulinal Toxin Produced by Different Stains of the Organism**
      - ✓ Type A toxin: most virulent; endospore most heat-resistant of all; usually proteolytic
      - ✓ Type B toxin: most European outbreaks and eastern United States; proteolytic and nonproteolytic
      - ✓ Type E toxin: involve seafood; endospore less heat-resistant (destroyed by boiling); nonproteolytic; can produce toxin at refrigerator temperatures
    - **Incidence and Treatment of Botulism**
      - ✓ Not a common disease; 50% Type A; problems arise due to food preparation methods; organism does not compete well with normal intestinal microbiota in adults, but infants may develop **infant botulism;** organism can grow in wounds causing **wound botulism;** treatment: no honey to infants under 1 year of age, antitoxins, respiratory assistance
      - ✓ **Botox:** the toxin of botulism has therapeutic uses: chronic headaches, cerebral palsy, Parkinson disease, multiple sclerosis, blepharospasm, strabismus, hyperhidrosis, cosmetic
- **Leprosy (Hansen's disease)**
  - *Mycobacterium leprae*: Acid fast positive (+) rods; optimum growth at 30° C; outer, cooler parts of the humans body; invades peripheral nervous system; cell damage due to cell-mediated immune response; inoculation of nude mice foot pads and armadillos used to culture; consist of **two forms**:
  - **Tuberculoid** (neural) **form: depigmented** regions of skin which have lost sensation, surrounded by border of nodules
  - **Lepromatous** (progressive) **form:** skin cells infected, disfiguring nodules form all over body; transfer of organism uncertain, possibly by nasal secretions and oozing material from lesions; cases in the United States increasing; treatment: sulfone drugs (dapsone), vaccines (BCG for tuberculosis)

C. Viral Diseases of the Nervous System
- **Poliomyelitis (Polio)**
  - *Poliovirus*: causes paralysis; most patients die due to respiratory muscle paralysis; mode of transmission is drinking contaminated water with feces containing the virus; multiplies in throat and small intestine; invades tonsils and lymph nodes, then enters blood →viremia; if persistent can enter CNS (primarily motor nerve cells in upper spinal cord); middle aged adults having polio as a child can develop **postpolio syndrome**
    - **Diagnosis:** by cell cultures and cytopathic effects
    - **Vaccine:** Three different serotypes of the poliovirus: Type 1, Type 2, Type 3; Two different vaccine types available
      - ✓ **Salk vaccine:** consist of all three Types, **inactivated**; called **inactivated polio vaccines (IPV)**
      - ✓ **Sabin vaccine:** contains living, **attenuated (weakened)** strains; ingested; also called **oral polio vaccine (OPV);** usually contains the three Types (trivalent, **tOPV**)
    - **Epidemiology and Eradication Efforts:** naturally occurring, wild-type virus (WPV) distinguished from vaccine-derived virus (VDPV); VDPV is an attenuated virus that reverted to virulence; WPV persist in some areas (Pakistan, India, Nigeria); also emergence of VDPV

- **Rabies**
  - *Rabies virus*: member of genus *Lyssavirus* (**ssRNA virus**); can result in fatal encephalitis; bullet shape; infected from bite of infected animal (dog, bat, skunk, fox, raccoon); proliferates in the PNS and travels to the CNS, enters salivary glands (increase salivation) and other organs; causes spasms of muscles of the mouth and pharynx; long incubation period; **furious (classic) rabies:** restless, highly excitable, snap at anything within reach; **paralytic (dumb or numb) rabies:** paralysis sets in, flow of saliva increases, swallowing more difficult, minimal excitability
    - **Diagnosis:** direct fluorescent-antibody test (**DFA**) which is extremely sensitive and specific, done on saliva or tissue biopsies; rapid immunohistochemical test (**RIT**)
    - **Prevention of Rabies:** high risk individuals (veterinarians, animal control workers, laboratory workers) vaccinated before exposure; if bitten one undergoes **postexposure prophylaxis (PEP):** series of antirabies vaccines (**human diploid cell vaccine (HDCV)**, or chick embryo-grown vaccines) and immunoglobulin (**human rabies immune globulin (RIG)**) injections
    - **Treatment of Rabies:** once symptomatic, little effective treatment; Milwaukee protocol
    - **Distribution of Rabies:** occurs all over the world
    - **Related *Lyssavirus* Encephalitis:** caused by genotypes of the genus *Lyssavirus* that are closely related to classic rabies virus; include: *Australian bat lyssavirus* (ABLV) and *European bat lyssavirus* (EBLV)
- **Arbovirus Encephalitis**
  - *Arbovirus*: short for **ar**thropod-**bo**rne virus; mosquito-borne viruses; incidence increase during summer months; include: chills, headache, fever, including death; horses and humans affected; strains: **eastern equine encephalitis (EEE), western equine encephalitis (WEE), St. Louis encephalitis (SLE), California encephalitis (CE), West Nile virus (WNV);** diagnosis based on serological test; control of mosquito vector most effective way to control encephalitis

D. Fungal Diseases of the Nervous System
- **Cryptococcus neoformans Meningitis**
  - *Cryptococcus neoformans*: causes **cryptococcosis**; well adapted to CNS fluid; form spherical cells resembling yeast; reproduce by budding; **polysaccharide capsule**; found in soil especially with infected pigeon/chicken droppings; along window ledges of urban buildings; transmitted by inhalation of droppings; hematologic spread especially in the immunocompromised; can result in progressive meningitis; **other species pathogenic to humans:** *Cryptococcus grubii and Cryptococcus gattii*; best diagnostic test: latex agglutination test to detect antigen; treatment: amphotericin B and flucytosine

E. Protozoan Diseases of the Nervous System
- **African Trypanosomiasis (or sleeping sickness)**
  - *Trypanosoma brucei*: causes sleeping sickness in humans; **two subspecies:** *Trypanosoma brucei gambiense* (humans only reservoir) and *Trypanosoma brucie rhodesiense* (parasite of domestic livestock and wild animals); carried by the **Tsetse fly**; are **flagellates;** once infected, few symptoms; chronic form of disease with fever, headaches, CNS deterioration; treatments: suramin, pentamidine, melarsoprol (toxic), eflornithine; control: attempt to eliminate vector tsetse fly
- **Amoebic Meningoencephalitis**
  - *Naegleria fowleri*: found in recreational freshwater (warm ponds or streams); causes **primary amebic meningoencephalitis (PAM);** victims are children; initially infects nasal mucosa, later the brain to grow; diagnosis made at autopsy; treatment amphotericin B

o *Granulomatous amebic encephalitis* (**GAE**): found in recreational freshwater; caused by a **species of Acanthamoeba;** chronic, slowly progressive, fatal; **granulomas** form; entry probably mucous membranes; lesions form in the brain, lungs, and other organs

G. Nervous System Diseases Caused by Prions
- The shape of the enzyme's protein component important for its operation
- Certain **normal proteins** are found on the surface of brain cell neurons; **function** of these **normal proteins** uncertain, but may influence maturation of nerve cells
- These **normal proteins** can assume two folded shapes: one normal, one abnormal
- If **normal** comes in contact with **abnormally folded protein (prion), normal changes it shape; becomes another prion;** leads to production of **new prions**
- Leads to clumping; forms aggregate of fibrils of misfolded proteins; aggregate→ neuronal cell death
- Autopsies show characteristic **spongiform degeneration** of the brain
- Study of these diseases called: **transmissible spongiform encephalopathies (TSE)**
- Typical **prion disease**
  o **Sheep scrapie:** in animals; will scrape itself until raw; gradually loses motor control and dies; disease spread to other animals by infection of brain tissue from one animal to next; seen also in mink; **chronic wasting disease:** affects deer, elk
  o **Classic Creutzfeldt-Jakob disease (CJD):** in humans; infection by corneal transplants and scalpel nicks during autopsy have been reported; traced to injection of growth hormone from human tissue; boiling, irradiation, autoclaving not reliable; sodium hydroxide and autoclaving at 134 °C recommended to sterilize; protease enzymes may be effective
  o **Kuru:** disease seen in some tribes in New Guinea; acquired through **cannibalic rituals**
  o **Bovine Spongiform Encephalopathy (BSE):** known as **mad cow disease;** origin ascribed to feed supplements contaminated with prions (sheep infected scrapie) **or** a spontaneous mutation in a cow; cattle eventually showed symptoms of **BSE;** only test is postmortem brain tissue; prevent introduction into the United States: prohibit use from "downer" animals, consumption of certain parts of cattle carcass
  o **Variant Creutsfeldt-Jakob Disease (vCJD):** variant of **classic CJD;** age at death (younger), duration of illness (longer than CJD), clinical presentation (delayed neurological signs, more psychiatric and behavioral), genotype differs (aa combinations)

H. Disease Caused by Unidentified Agents
- **Chronic Fatigue Syndrome:** also **called myalgic encephalomyelitis (ME);** one complains of **persistent fatigue which is debilitating;** multiple allergies; person does not cope well with stresses; prone to infections; continues for months or years; linked to immune system; may have a genetic component; more common in women; no treatment

MICROBIOLOGY

MICROBIAL DISEASES OF THE RESPIRATORY SYSTEM

A. Structure and Function of the Respiratory System
- **Upper respiratory system:** consists of nose, pharynx, middle ear, eustachian tubes
- **Lower respiratory system:** larynx, trachea, bronchial tubes, **alveoli**
  - **Alveoli:** oxygen and carbon dioxide exchanged

B. Normal Microbiota of the Respiratory System
- Upper respiratory system: potential pathogenic microorganisms make up part of the normal microbiota; usually do not cause disease
- Lower respiratory system: nearly sterile

C. Microbial Diseases of the Upper Respiratory System
- **Pharyngitis:** inflammation of mucous membranes involving the throat
- **Laryngitis:** inflammation of the larynx
- **Tonsillitis:** inflammation of tonsils
- **Sinusitis:** inflammation of the sinus
- **Epiglottitis:** inflammation of the epiglottis
- **Bacterial Diseases of the Upper Respiratory System**
  - **Streptococcal Pharyngitis (Strep Throat):** caused by gram positive (+) group A streptococci (**GAS**), solely of *Streptococcus pyogenes*; pathogenicity of **GAS** due to: resistant to phagocytes, produce **streptokinase** and **streptolysins;** transmitted by respiratory secretions; one sees local inflammation of the throat, fever; tonsillitis and otitis media can occur; diagnosed by enzyme immunoassay (**EIA**); treatment: penicillin
  - **Scarlet Fever:** cause by *Streptococcus pyogenes* strain producing an **erythrogenic toxin; toxin** produces a pinkish red skin rash; tongue has a spotted **strawberry-like appearance;** relatively rare and mild disease
  - **Diphtheria:** caused by *Corynebacterium diphtheriae*; gram positive (+) pleomorphic, club shaped rod; part of the normal immunization for children, **DTaP vaccine;** transmitted airborne; tough grayish membrane in throat causing swelling; some strains releases an **exotoxin;** treatment: diphtheria toxoid (**Td**), penicillin, erythromycin
    - **Cutaneous diphtheria**: infects skin, usually at wound site, with minimal systemic circulation of the toxin
  - **Otitis Media:** infection of the middle ear; common in children; **most common pathogen** is *Streptococcus pneumoniae*; other causes: *Haemophilus influenzae, Streptococcus pyogenes, Moraxella catarrhalis, Staphylococcus aureus*; pus formation→painful ear ache; treatment: amoxicillin, conjugate vaccine
- **Viral Diseases of the Upper Respiratory System**
  - **The Common Cold:** hundreds of different viruses causing the common cold (**rhinovirus,** coronaviruses); symptoms include: sneezing, nasal secretions, congestion; infection can spread
    - **Rhinoviruses: most common:** carried on airborne droplets; transmitted by sneezing, coughing, person to person contact; treat symptoms: cough suppressant, antihistamines

D. Microbial Diseases of the Lower Respiratory System
- Caused by many bacteria and viruses causing upper respiratory infections
- **Bronchitis:** inflammation of the bronchi
- **Bronchiolitis:** inflammation of the bronchioles
- **Pneumonia:** pulmonary alveoli involved
- **Bacterial Diseases of the Lower Respiratory System**
  - **Pertussi (Whooping Cough):** caused by *Bordetella pertussis*; obligately aerobic gram negative (-) coccobacillus; virulent stain has **capsule**; attach to ciliated cells in the trachea; produces **toxins: tracheal cytotoxin, pertussis toxin**; primarily a childhood disease; stages of disease: initial stage (**catarrhal stage,** symptoms like common cold), second stage (**paroxysmal stage,** prolonged episodes of coughing), third state **convalescense stage** (healing); gasping for air causes whooping sound; treatment: DTaP vaccine, erythromycin, macrolides
  - **Tuberculosis (TB):** caused by *Mycobacterium tuberculosis*; rod shaped, **acid fast** positive (+); acquired by inhalation, phagocytized by macrophages in the alveoli; if progression continues, leads to **tubercle** formation; when disease is arrested, lesions heal, becoming calcified (**Ghon's complexes**); if body's defenses poor, disease can spread in blood (**miliary tuberculosis**) to other organs; diagnosis: **tuberculin skin test, mantoux,** sputum smears, PCR methods; treatment (minimum of (6) **six months** of therapy): **first line drugs:** combination of isoniazid, rifampicin, ethambutol, pyrazinamide), **second line drugs:** several aminoglycosides, fluoroquinolones, para-aminosalicylic acid (**PAS**); streptomycin still used; for **multi-drug-resistant (MDR)** and **extensively drug-resistant (XDR)** strains, effective drugs being investigated; vaccines: **BCG;** testing for drug susceptibility can take months for final results;
    - *Mycobacterium bovine*: causes **bovine tuberculosis**; pathogen of cattle; transmitted to humans via contaminated milk or food; affects bones or lymphatic system
    - *Mycobacterium avium-intracellulare*: seen in late stages of HIV infection
- **Bacterial Pneumonias**
  - **Typical** (*Streptococcus pneumoniae*) versus **Atypical** (fungi, viruses, protozoa, mycoplasma)
  - Pneumonias named after part of lower respiratory area that is affected: **Lobar** (lobes involved), **Broncho** (alveoli of the lungs next to bronchi infected), **Pleurisy** (pleural membranes inflamed)
    - **Pneumococcal Pneumonia:** caused by *Streptococcus Pneumoniae*; gram positive (+), cocci or ovoid in shape; usually in pairs; **dense capsule;** involves both the bronchi and alveoli; symptoms are: high fever, breathing difficulty, chest pain; **sputum is rust-colored** from blood; diagnosis from throat, sputum, other fluids; diagnosis: **optochin test** (zone of inhibition present), bile solubility test; treatment: penicillin, fluoroquinolones, macrolides, vaccines
    - **Haemophilus influenzae pneumonia:** caused by *Haemophilus influenzae*; gram negative (-) coccobacillus; alcoholics, poor nutrition, diabetics, cancer patients very susceptible; diagnosed using special media (contains **X** and **Y** factors); treatment: second generation cephalosporins
    - **Mycoplasmal pneumonia (Atypical or Walking):** caused by *Mycoplasma pneumonia:* does not have cell wall; common in children and young adults; symptoms: low grade fever, cough, headache for several weeks; **"fried egg"** appearance on medium; diagnosis: PCR and serological tests; treatment: tetracycline (for symptoms)
    - **Legionellosis (Legionnaires' Disease):** caused by *Legionella pneumophila*; gram negative(-) rod; exist in **biofilm;** replicates within macrophages; grows: in water of air conditioning cooling towers, hospital water lines, humidifiers, whirlpools; symptoms: high fever, cough, general symptoms of pneumonia; men over 50 years of age; smokers, alcoholics; diagnosis: **charcoal-yeast extract** medium, fluorescent-antibody methods, DNA probe test; treatment: erythromycin, azithromycin

- ✓ **Pontiac fever:** caused by *Legionella pneumophila*; another form of **legionellosis;** symptoms include: fever, muscle aches, cough; self-limiting
  - **Psittacosis (Ornithosis):** caused by *Chlamydophila psittaci*; gram negative (-) obligate intracellular bacteria; form tiny **elementary bodies;** associated with birds (parakeets, pigeons, ducks, chickens, parrots); transmission to humans by birds (birds have: diarrhea, ruffled feathers, respiratory illness); symptoms: fever, coughing, chills, headache; diagnosed: embryonated eggs or cell culture, serological tests; treatment: tetracycline; no vaccine
  - **Chlamydial Pneumonia:** caused by *Chlamydophila pneumoniae*; common in college students; clinically resembles mycoplasmal pneumonia; treatment: tetracycline
  - **Q Fever:** caused by *Coxiella burnetii*; obligate intracellular parasitic bacterium; parasite of several arthropods (ticks); transmitted among animals by tick bites; spread to humans ingesting unpasteurized milk or inhaling aerosols of microbes; range of symptoms: **acute Q fever** (fever, headaches, muscle aches, coughing, malaise) and **chronic Q fever** (endocarditis); diagnosis: chick embryos or cell cultures; treatment: doxycycline with chloroquine
  - **Melioidosis:** caused by *Burkholderia pseudomallei*; gram negative (-) rod; organism widely distributed in moist soils; affects individuals with low immune capabilities; common in southeast Asia and northern Australia; clinically looks like pneumonia; can cause necrotizing fasciitis, encephalitis; transmission primarily by inhalation, inoculation through puncture wounds; treatment: ceftazidime

E. Viral Diseases of the Lower Respiratory System
- Many respiratory illnesses caused by viruses
- The **xTAG respiratory panel:** new test to help diagnose numerous illnesses at a time
  - **Viral Pneumonia:** can occur as a complication of chicken pox, influenza, measles
  - **Respiratory Syncytial Virus (RSV):** most common cause in infants (2 to 6 months of age); also seen in the elderly; common in winter and early spring; symptoms: coughing, wheezing for more than a week; serological testing done; cause cell fusion when grown in cell culture; treatment: immune globulin product, vaccines being tested, aerosol ribavin (antiviral drug), humanized monoclonal antibody palivizumab (Synagis)
  - **Influenza (Flu):** symptoms: chills, fever, headache, muscular aches
    - **The Influenza Virus:** viruses in the genus *Influenzavirus*: consist of 8 separate **RNA segments**, enclosed by inner layer of **protein** and **an outer lipid bilayer;** numerous projections embedded in **bilayer;** two types of projections: **hemagglutinin (HA) spikes** and **neuraminidase (NA) spikes; HA:** for attachment to cells; **NA:** enzyme used to help virus to separate from infected cell and stimulate formation of antibodies; viral strains identified by **variation** in **HA** and **NA** antigens; (there are 16 subtypes of **HA** and 9 of **NA); variations** determined by:
      - ✓ **Antigenic drift: high mutation rates**, due to lack of proofreading ability, allow virus to evade host immunity
      - ✓ **Antigenic shifts:** involve genetic recombination (**reassortment**) involving the 8 RNA segments
    - **Epidemiology of Influenza:** every year, epidemics spread through large populations; most recent pandemic in 2009, involving **H1N1 virus;** strain circulating in pigs (swine); mutated in humans
    - The virus occurs in avian and mammalian strains; humans generally not affected by avian strains
    - **Influenza Vaccines:** ones used are **multivalent**; two types of vaccines available: injected inactivated version **and** nasal spray made with live attenuated virus

- **The 1918-1919 Pandemic: 20-50 million people died**
- **Diagnosis of Influenza:** difficult to isolate
- **Treatment:** with amantadine, rimantadine, zanamivir (Relenza) inhaled, oseltamivir (Tamiflu) oral

F. Fungal Diseases of the Lower Respiratory System

- Fungi often produce spores that spread through the air
- Opportunistic fungi grow in immunosuppressed, immunocompromised, transplant patients, AIDS
  - **Histoplasmosis:** caused *by Histoplasma capsulatum*; **dimorphic fungus** (yeast-like shape in tissue, and filamentous form in soil or artificial media); found intracellularly in macrophages; can spread from lungs to other organs; geographically located in states adjoining the Ohio and Mississippi rivers; symptoms: poorly defined, can become severe; acquired airborne, bird and bat droppings; diagnosis: serological tests, DNA probes; treatment: amphotericin B, itraconazole
  - **Coccidioidomycosis:** caused by *Coccidioides immitis*; **dimorphic fungus** (**spherule** filled with endospores in tissue; filamentous in soil); found in dry alkaline soils of American southwest, South America and northern Mexico; also known as Valley Fever or San Joaquin fever; spread by wind; symptoms: chest pain, fever, coughing, weight loss; diagnosis: identifying spherules, serological tests, DNA probes; treatment: amphotericin B, ketoconazole, itraconazole
  - **Pneumocystis pneumonia:** caused by *Pneumocystis jirovecii* (formerly *Pneumocystis carinii*); characteristics of both fungus and protozoan; infants and persons immunocompromised susceptible (AIDS, cancer patients); found in lining of alveoli; diagnosis: cysts in sputum samples; treatment: trimethoprim-sulfamethoxazole, clindamycin, IV pentamidine
  - **Blastomycosis (North American Blastomycosis):** caused by *Blastomyces dermatitidis*; **dimorphic fungus**; Mississippi and Ohio River valleys; grows in soil; symptoms: resembles bacterial pneumonia, cutaneous ulcers, abscess formation and tissue damage; diagnosis: pus and tissue biopsy; treatment: amphotericin B, itraconazole
  - **Aspergillosis:** caused by *Aspergillus fumigatus*; airborne; grows well in compost piles; farmers and gardeners most often exposed
  - *Rhizopus and Mucor*: spore producers

MICROBIOLOGY

MICROBIAL DISEASES OF THE URINARY AND REPRODUCTIVE SYSTEM

A. Structure and Function of the Urinary System
- Consists of two: kidneys, ureters; one: urinary bladder, urethra
- Regulates the chemical composition and volume of the blood; excretes nitrogenous waste and water

B. Structure and Function of the Reproductive System
- Female: consists of two: ovaries, fallopian tubes; one uterus (includes cervix), vagina, external genitals)
- Male: two testes; system of ducts, accessory glands, penis
- Both: produce gametes and hormones

C. Normal Microbiota of the Urinary and Reproductive Systems
- Female and male **urinary systems**: normal **urine is sterile;** may become contaminated by microbes on the skin
- Female **reproductive system** (in vagina): lactobacilli, streptococcus, various anaerobes, some gram negative (-), *Candida albicans*
- Male **reproductive system** (urethra): usually sterile, except for few contaminating microbes near external orifice

D. Diseases of the Urinary System
- **Bacterial Diseases of the Urinary System**
- Forms of **Inflammation**
  - o **Urethritis**: inflammation of the urethra
  - o **Cystitis**: inflammation of the bladder
  - o **Ureteritis**: inflammation of the ureters
  - o **Pyelonephritis**: inflammation of the kidneys
- **Cystitis:** very common in females; symptoms: dysuria and pyuria; most cases due to *Escherichia coli* (identified on **MacConkey's agar**), followed by *Staphylococcus saprophyticus*; diagnosis: urine sample, test **for leukocyte esterase (LE)** indicates active infection; treatment: ampicillin, trimethoprim-sulfamethoxazole, fluoroquinolone
- **Pyelonephritis:** involves one or both kidneys; often due to progression of cystitis; can result into bacteremia; symptoms: fever, flank or back pain; can become chronic, scarring kidneys; most cases due to *Escherichia coli*; diagnosis: **Gram stain** (of urine), blood cultures; treatment: intravenous broad spectrum antibiotics
- **Leptospirosis:** disease of domestic or wild animals, passed to humans; can cause kidney or liver damage (**Weil's disease**); an emerging form affects the lungs (**pulmonary hemorrhagic syndrome**) caused by *Leptospira interrogans*: tighly wound spirochete, **obligate aerobic;** can grow in artificial media supplemented with rabbit serum; transmission: from urine of infected animal, to humans by contact with urine contaminated water; symptoms: headaches, muscle aches, chills, fever; diagnosis: serological test, blood, urine, or other fluids for the microbe of its DNA; treatment: doxycycline

E. Diseases of the Reproductive Systems
- Microbes causing infections requires intimate contact for transmission
- **Bacterial Diseases of the Reproductive Systems**
  - Most transmitted by sexual activity called **sexually transmitted diseases (STDs)**
  - Movement to replace terminology with **sexually transmitted infections (STIs)**
  - **Gonorrhea:** caused by gram negative (-) diplococcus *Neisseria gonorrhoeae*; **fimbriae**
    - Attaches and penetrates mucosal epithelial cells; inflammation leading to pus formation
    - Symptoms: **males** (painful urination, pus discharge, urethritis, epididymitis, blockage of the urethra and sterility); **females** (disease is more insidious, cervix infected, abdominal pain, PID, sterility); **both sexes** can develop systemic complications (involving joints, heart, meninges, eyes, other parts); **pregnant woman** (eyes of infant can be infected passing through birth canal, resulting in blindness (called **ophthalmia neonatorum**); **pharyngeal gonorrhea** (resembles septic sore throat); and **anal gonorrhea** (painful, discharge, itching)
    - Diagnosis: **males** (gram stain on smear of pus from urethra); **female** (sample from cervix taken and grown on special media); **both sexes:** ELISA, monoclonal antibodies against antigens on surface of the pathogen, nucleic acid amplification tests
    - Treatment: cefixime, ceftriaxone (gonorrhea affecting cervical, urethral, rectal tissues); ceftriaxone (pharyngeal infection); doxycycline (for **coinfection** by *Chlamydia trachomatis*); also treat **sex partners** of patient
  - **Nongonococcal Urethritis (NGU):** also known as **nonspecific urethritis (NSU)**; any inflammation of the urethra **not caused by** *Neisseria gonorrhoeae*
    - Most common cause by *Chlamydia trachomatis* (sometimes coinfects with gonorrhea)
    - *Chlamydia trachomatis* also responsible for the **STI lymphogranuloma venereum**
    - Symptoms: usually asymptomatic; **both sexes** experience painful urination, watery discharge; **males** (epididymitis); **females** (PID, sterility, increased risk of cervical cancer); **infected mothers** (eye infections, pneumonia in infants)
    - Diagnosis: best done by specialized cultivation methods; non-culture-based tests: detect DNA or RNA sequences, urine samples
    - **Other bacteria implicated in NGU:** *Ureaplasma urealyticum* (cause: urethritis, infertility) *Mycoplasma hominis* (inhabits normal vagina, opportunistically can cause fallopian tube infection)
  - **Pelvic Inflammatory Disease (PID):** collective term for extensive bacterial infection of the female pelvic organs; can lead to chronic pain or infertility
    - A **polymicrobial** disease: many different pathogens might be the cause, including coinfections
    - Complications of **PID: Salpingitis** (infection of the fallopian tubes), **ectopic pregnancy:** fertilized egg implants outside the uterus, can lead to rupture of tube, hemorrhage
    - Diagnosis: signs and symptoms, laboratory test, ultrasound
    - Treatment: doxycycline and cefoxitin
  - **Syphilis:** caused by *Treponema pallidum*; a gram negative (-), motile, thin, tightly coiled spirochete
    - Relies on host for many compounds needed for life; propagated in rabbits; can grow in cell cultures at low oxygen concentrations, but for a few generations; produces several lipoproteins that induce an inflammatory immune response
    - Separate strains (*Treponema pallidum pertenue*) responsible for tropical endemic skin diseases (**yaws**); not sexually transmitted
    - Transmitted by sexual contact, of all kinds; **disease progresses through several stages**

- ✓ **Primary stage**: small, painless, hard-based ulceration (**chancre**) at site of infection; an exudate of serum forms in the center containing many spirochetes; lesion disappears in a few weeks; bacteria entering bloodstream and lymphatics
- ✓ **Secondary stage**: rashes on skin, mucous membranes, palms and soles (due to inflammatory response to circulating immune complexes lodging in various body sites); patches of hair loss; malaise, fever; considered **the infectious stage (transmission occurs during primary and secondary stage);** symptoms resolve within 3 months
- ✓ **Latent period**: no symptoms; after 2 to 4 years, disease not normally infectious (except transmission from mother to fetus); majority of cases do not progress beyond the latent period
- ✓ **Tertiary stage**: disease reappears; most symptoms probably due to body's immune reaction to surviving spirochetes; characterized by gummas (**gummatous syphilis**) which are **rubbery masses** located in various organs, causing tissue destruction; **Cardiovascular syphilis** (weakening of the aorta); **Neurosyphilis** (affects CNS: personality changes, dementia, seizures, partial paralysis, loss of hearing or sight, loss of speech, loss of bladder control)

- ■ **Congenital syphilis**: crosses placenta to unborn fetus; leads to neurological damage; stillbirth
- ■ **Diagnosis of Syphilis**: complex due to stages of the disease; tests fall into **three groups**: visual microscopic, nontreponemal serological test, and treponemal serological test (FTA-ABS)
  - ✓ **Visual Microscopic**: important for screening for **primary syphilis**; spirochete can be detected in exudates of lesions by **darkfield** microscopy, or direct fluorescent-antibody test (**DFA-TP**)
  - ✓ **Nontreponemal Serological Test**: at **secondary stage**, serological test are reactive; test detects **reagin-type antibodies** (antibodies which are a response to lipid materials the body forms as an indirect reaction to infection by the spirochete); the **antigen used** is an extract of beef heart (**cardiolipin**) containing lipids similar to those that stimulate the **reagin-type antibodies;** tests: **VDRL** (Venereal Disease Research Laboratory)**test, RPR** (rapid plasma reagin) **test, ELISA test** using the VDLR antigen
  - ✓ **Treponemal-type Serological Test**: used for **confirmatory testing;** react **directly with the spirochete;** tests: **EIA (enzyme immunoassay)** treponemal tests, **RDTs (rapid diagnostic tests); FTA-ABS (fluorescent treponemal antibody absorption)** test is an **indirect fluorescent –antibody test**
- ■ Treatment : Benzathine penicillin, tetracycline, azithromycin, doxycycline
- o **Lymphogranuloma Venereum (LV):** uncommon in the United States, common in tropical regions
  - ■ Caused by *Chlamydia trachomatis*; invades lymphatic system; lymph nodes become enlarged, tender; inflammation can result in scarring which obstructs lymph vessels
  - ■ Diagnosis: blood test for antibodies; grows in cell culture or embryonated egg
  - ■ Treatment: doxycycline
- o **Chancroid (Soft Chancre):** occurs most frequently in tropical areas
  - ■ Caused by *Haemophilus ducreyi*; gram positive (+) rod; symptoms: swollen, painful ulcer forms on genitals; infected lymph nodes may discharge pus to surface; diagnosis: culture of bacteria; treatment: erythromycin, ceftriaxone
- o **Bacterial Vaginosis:** caused by *Gardnerella vaginalis*; small, pleomorphic, gram -variable rod
  - ■ Precipitated by changes in vagina causing imbalance between normal bacterial flora; decrease in numbers of *Lactobacillus* leads to increase in *Gardnerella vaginalis*; changes vaginal pH (above 4.5); symptoms: vaginal pH > 4.5, frothy discharge; premature and low birth weight infants

- Diagnosis: **'fishy odor'** (**whiff test**) when tested with potassium hydroxide, **clue cells** (epithelial cells covered by bacteria; treatment: metronidazole

- **Viral Diseases of the Reproductive Systems**
  - Very difficult to treat
  - **Genital Herpes:** usually caused by *herpes simplex virus type 2* (**HSV-2**) also named **HHV-2**
    - Infection acquired by oral-genital contact; symptoms: lesions cause burning/tingling sensation followed by vesicles, painful urination and walking; vesicles heal
    - Vesicles contain infectious fluid; recurs often; reactivation due to several factors: stress, menses
    - Diagnosis: culture virus from vesicles, PCR, serological tests. treatment: no cure; acyclovir, famciclovir, valacyclovir
    - **Neonatal Herpes:** virus crosses placental barrier and affects the fetus; can cause: spontaneous abortion, mental retardation, vision and hearing defects; diagnose: fluorescent antibody tests, PCR test; treatment: no vaccine currently, intravenous administration of acyclovir
  - **Genital Warts:** caused by papillomaviruses (**HPV**); greater than 60 types of **HPV, genital warts** (**condyloma acuminate**) transmitted sexually; **warty appearance**
    - Visible genital warts caused by serotypes **6 and 11**; serotypes **16 and 18** associated with causing **cancer** (cervical, oral, anal, penile); treatment: vaccines (Gardasil, Cervarix), methods: surgery, cryotherapy, gels (podofilix, imiquimod), Imiquimod (Aldara)
  - **AIDS:** or **HIV** infections; pathogenicity based on damage to immune system
- **Fungal Diseases of the Reproductive Systems**
  - **Candidiasis:** caused most commonly by *Candida albicans* (85% - 90%); *Candida glabrata*
    - Results from opportunistic overgrowth when normal microbiota are suppressed by antibiotics
    - Symptoms of vulvovaginal candidiasis: thick, yellow, cheesy discharge, severe itching, yeasty odor; predisposing conditions: oral contraceptives, pregnancy, diabetes, antibiotics
    - Diagnosis: fungus in scrapings by microscopy, isolation in culture; treatment: clotrimazole, miconazole, fluconazole
- **Protozoan Diseases of the Reproductive Systems**
  - Affects young, sexually active women; **may be most common STD/STI**
  - **Trichomoniasis:** caused by *Trichomonas vaginalis*; normal inhabitant of the vagina
    - Overgrowth when normal acidity of vagina is disturbed; symptoms: greenish yellow discharge with foul odor, irritation and itching; men rarely have symptoms; known to cause preterm delivery and low birth weight
    - Diagnosis: organisms in discharge seen by microscopy, grown on media, DNA probes, monoclonal antibodies; treatment: metronidazole (both partners)
- **TORCH Panel of Tests**
  - **TORCH** is an acronym for a panel of tests used in screening antibodies for infections
    - **T**oxoplasma
    - **O**ther (syphilis, hepatitis B, enterovirus, Epstein-Barr virus, varicella-zoster virus)
    - **R**ubella
    - **C**ytomegalovirus
    - **H**erpes simplex virus

MICROBIOLOGY

MICROBIAL DISEASES OF THE DIGESTIVE SYSTEM

A. Structure and Function of the Digestive System
- Purpose is to digest foods (break down, absorb, eliminate)
- A tube-like structure: mainly mouth, pharynx, esophagus, stomach, small and large, rectum, anus
- Includes accessory structures: teeth, tongue, salivary glands, liver, gallbladder, pancreas
- Relationship between digestive system and the immune system

B. Normal Microbiota of the Digestive System
- Bacteria populate the mouth, saliva, large intestine (**anaerobics and facultative anaerobics**)
- Stomach and small intestine have few microbes

C. Bacterial Diseases of the Mouth
- **Dental Caries (Tooth Decay)**
  - Caused by **dental plaque**: type of **biofilm**; an accumulation of microbes and their products; involved in production of **dental caries**; over 700 species of bacteria identified in oral cavity; **most important cariogenic bacterium** is
    - *Streptococcus mutans*: gram positive (+) cocci; metabolizes large range of carbohydrates, tolerates acidity, synthesizes **dextran**
    - Initiation of **caries**: depends on the attachment of *Streptococcus mutans* to tooth; bacteria adhere to tooth coated with thin film of proteins (pellicle) from saliva→**cariogenic bacteria** attach and produce **dextran** (product by the hydrolysis of sucrose into glucose and fructose); glucose molecule assembled into dextran by **the enzyme glucosyltransferase**; residual fructose fermented into lactic acid→**caries**→abscess formation
  - Other species of *Streptococcus* are also **cariogenic**
  - **Bacterial population of plaque** can have over 400 bacterial species (predominately *Streptococci* and *Actinomyces*)
  - Older **calcified plaque** called **tartar**
  - Sugar alcohols (mannitol, sorbitol, xylitol) **are not cariogenic**
  - Prevention: minimum intake of sucrose, brushing, flossing, professional cleaning, use of fluoride, mouthwash (chlorhexidine)
- **Periodontal Disease**
  - Caused by inflammation and degeneration of structures that support the teeth
  - Roots of teeth protected by **cementum**
    - **Gingivitis**: inflammation restricted to the gums (**gingivae**); bleeding of gums while brushing teeth; caused by: Streptococci, Actinomycetes, anaerobic gram negative (-) bacteria
    - **Periodontitis**: progression of **chronic gingivitis**; gums inflamed and bleed easily; pus, bone, and tissue supporting teeth destroyed→loosening or loss of teeth; primarily caused by *Porphyromonas* species; treated surgically
    - **Acute necrotizing ulcerative gingivitis (Vincent's disease/trench mouth)**: bacteria associated is *Prevotella intermedia*; **anaerobic**: painful during chewing; **halitosis**; treatment with oxidizing agents, debridement, metronidazole

D. Bacterial Diseases of the Lower Digestive System

- Diseases are of two types: **Infections** and **Intoxications**
    - o **Infections:** microbes enters, penetrate, multiplies in GI tract; **M cells** translocate microbes and antigens to other side of epithelial lining; translocation causes contact of the antigen or microbe with lymphoid tissues; this initiates an immune response; **infection** characterized by: delay in GI symptoms, usually fever
    - o **Intoxication:** cause disease by forming **toxins; intoxication** caused by ingestion of a preformed toxin; **intoxication** characterized by: sudden appearance (within 1 hour) of GI symptoms, fever is less often
    - o **Infections** and **Intoxication**: both often cause: **diarrhea, dysentery** (diarrhea with mucus and/ or blood), abdominal cramping, nausea, vomiting; treatment: fluid and electrolyte replacement
    - o **Gastroenteritis** (inflammation of the stomach and intestinal mucosa)
- **Staphylococcal Food Poisoning (Staphylococcal Enterotoxicosis)**
    - o Leading cause of gastroenteritis; caused by ingesting an **enterotoxin** produced by *Staphylococcus aureus*; **highly resistant** to: environmental stresses, heat, drying out, radiation, high osmotic pressures; often an inhabitant on the nasal passage (can contaminates hands)**,** cause of skin lesions; contaminates foods; if incubation in food (called **temperature abuse**), will reproduce and release **enterotoxin;** this **toxin is: heat stable**, can withstand boiling up to 30 minutes
    - o *Staphylococcus aureus*: produces several toxins which damage tissue and aid in virulence; a **superantigen**
    - o Toxin produced by Serological Type A often associated to the production of enzyme **coagulase** (coagulates blood plasma), described as **coagulase-positive**
    - o Growth facilitated if competing microbes in food are eliminated
    - o High risk foods include: custards, ham, cream pies, poultry; foods need to be kept refrigerated
    - o Symptoms: abdominal cramps, diarrhea within a few hours; diagnosis: based on symptoms, **phage typing**; pathogenic *Staphylococcus*: usually ferment **mannitol**, produce **hemolysins** and **coagulase**, form **yellow colonies**
- **Shigellosis (Bacillary Dysentery)**
    - o Caused by a group of **facultative anaerobic** gram negative (-)rods of the genus *Shigella*; not affected much by stomach acidity; attach to **M cells** which take bacterium into cell; bacteria multiply within cell; spread to neighboring cell producing **shiga toxin** (usually virulent) destroying tissue; rarely spread into bloodstream; dysentery is result of intestinal wall damage
    - o Four species that are pathogenic: *Shigella sonnei, Shigella dysenteriae, Shigella flexneri, Shigella boydii*; reside in intestinal tract of humans, apes, monkeys
    - o In United States, *Shigella sonnei*, most common species; causes mild dysentery
    - o Severe dysentery and prostration caused by *Shigella dysenteriae*
    - o Additional symptoms: abdominal cramps, fever; diagnosis: recovery of microbes by rectal swabs; treatment: fluoroquinolones, hydration
- **Salmonellosis (*Salmonella* Gastroenteritis)**
    - o Caused by **many** *Salmonella enterica* serovars: gram negative (-), **facultative anaerobic non-endospore forming** rods; normal inhabitant of the **intestine in humans and animals** (chickens, eggs, pet reptiles); all considered pathogenic; cause **salmonellosis**
    - o Salmonellae pathologically divided into **nontyphoidal salmonellae** (milder disease of salmonellosis) and **typhoidal salmonellae**
    - o Invade intestinal mucosa; multiply in vesicles inside epithelial cells; leads to inflammation; occasionally enter blood stream and lymphatics →many organs; symptoms: fever, nausea, abdominal cramps, diarrhea; diagnosis: isolating organism in stool or leftover foods, PCR tests; treatment: oral rehydration; prevent: good sanitation practices

- **Typhoid Fever**
  - o Caused by *Salmonella typhi* (**most virulent serotype**); **found only in humans**; spread in human feces; prevalent in other parts of the world; multiply within phagocytic cells; disseminate to multiple organs (liver, spleen); phagocytic cells lyse and release pathogen into bloodstream; symptoms: high fever, headaches, diarrhea, ulceration of intestinal wall associated with poor sanitation
  - o Number of recovered patients become **chronic carriers,** where pathogen grows and multiples in gallbladder; treatment: chloramphenicol, quinolones or third-generation cephalosporins, vaccines
- **Cholera**
  - o Caused by *Vibrio cholerae*; slightly curved, gram negative (-) rod, single polar flagellum; form biofilms; grow in small intestine; produce **exotoxin cholera toxin**: causes host cells to secretes water and electrolytes, especially potassium; results in **"rice water stools"** (up to 5 gallons of fluid lost), vomiting; adapt to **salty contaminated waters**; diagnosed: symptoms and cultures from feces
  - o Sensitive to stomach acids
  - o Serogroups **O:1** and **O:139**: both produce **exotoxin** which alters intestinal membrane permeability; lead to vomiting and diarrhea
  - o Treatment: doxycycline, replacement of fluids and electrolytes
- **Noncholera Vibrios**
  - o *Vibrio parahaemolyticus*: found in **salt water estuaries** in parts of the world; requires sodium and high osmotic pressure for growth; associated with raw oysters, shrimp, crabs; symptoms: resemble cholera, but milder; treatment: antibiotics and rehydration
  - o *Vibrio vulnificus*: found in **estuaries**; **halophilic** and requires sodium chloride for growth; also associated with eating of raw oyster, shrimps, crabs
- *Escherichia coli* **Gastroenteritis**
  - o *Escherichia coli*: in human intestinal tract; common and easily cultivated
  - o Normally harmless, but certain strains pathogenic
  - o Some **toxin-secreting pathogenic strains** able to invade intestinal epithelial cells causing *E. coli gastroenteritis*
  - o Can affect other locations: urinary tract, bloodstream, central nervous system
  - o Several pathogenic varieties (**pathovars**) have been identified
    - ■ **Enteropathogenic *E. coli* (EPEC)**: major cause of diarrhea in developing countries, fatal in infants; attach to intestinal wall, destroy the microvilli, form **actin rich pedestal-like projections**; secrete proteins which are translocated into host cell; some proteins contribute to diarrhea
    - ■ **Enteroinvasive *E. coli* (EIEC)**: same pathogenic mechanisms as *Shigella*; through **M** cells, gains access to the submucosa of intestinal tract; results: inflammation, fever, *Shigella*-**like dysentery**
    - ■ **Enteroaggregate *E. coli* (EAEC)**: group of coliforms found **only in humans**; on tissue culture cells, bacteria cause a **"stacked-brick"** configuration; not invasive; produce an **enterotoxin** causing watery diarrhea
    - ■ **Enterohemorrhagic *E. coli* (EHEC)**: sometimes called **Shiga-toxin-producing *E. coli* (STEC)**; same **pedestal** formation as **EPEC**; virulence factor is **shiga toxin**; most outbreaks due to **EHEC O157:H7**; toxin released when cell is lysed; **cattle main reservoir**; infection spread by contaminated water or food; in humans, **shiga toxins**: often causes self-limiting diarrhea, but can produce **hemorrhagic colitis**; EHEC release the toxin into the lumen of the intestine; do not invade intestinal wall; EHEC also causes **hemolytic uremic syndrome (HUS):** blood in urine, kidney failure; treatment: rehydration, monitoring

electrolytes, dialysis, transplant; diagnosis: selective and differential media (**sorbitol-pathogen unable to ferment sorbitol**), **pulsed-field gel electrophoresis (PFGE)**; vaccines for cattle

- ■ **Enterotoxigenic *E. coli* (ETEC):** secretes **enterotoxins** (one resembles the **cholera toxin** in its function) which cause diarrhea; fatal for children under 5 years of age; **ETEC** not invasive and remain in lumen of the intestine
- ■ **Traveler's Diarrhea (TD): most common** bacterial cause is **ETEC**; second is **EAEC**; **TD** caused by other pathogens: *Salmonella, Shigella, Campylobacter,* viruses, protozoan parasites; treatment: usually oral rehydration, antimicrobial drugs (extreme cases) antibiotics, bismuth-containing preparations (Pepto- Bismol)

- ● *Campylobacter* **Gastroenteritis**
  - o Millions of cases caused by *Campylobacter jejuni,* in the United States; gram negative (-), **microaerophilic**, spiral curved bacteria; adapt well in intestines of animals **(especially poultry)**; culturing requires conditions of **low oxygen** and **high carbon dioxide**; optimum growth temperature 42 °C; almost all retail chicken contaminated; excreted in feces and milk of cattle; symptoms: fever, abdominal cramping, diarrhea or dysentery
  - o The infection linked to **Guillain-Barre syndrome** (a temporary paralysis)

- ● *Helicobacter* **Peptic Ulcer Disease**
  - o Caused by *Helicobacter pylori*; spiral shaped **microaerophilic** bacterium; responsible for most cases of **peptic ulcer disease (PUD);** inflammation→ ulceration; includes gastric and duodenal ulcers; persons of **Type O blood** more susceptible; considered a **carcinogenic bacterium** (gastric cancer can develop); *Helicobacter pylori* grow well in **highly acidic** environment of the stomach; produces large amounts of **urease** (converts **urea** to alkaline compound **ammonia**), causing a high pH in areas of growth; treatment: antibiotics, Bismuth subsalicylate (Pepto-Bismol), antibiotics; reinfection can result; diagnostic test: biopsy of tissue, culture, urea breath test, stool samples

- ● *Yersinia* **Gastroenteritis (Yersiniosis)**
  - o Caused by *Yersinia enterocolitica* and *Yersinia pseudotuberculosis*; **both:** gram negative (-); intestinal inhabitants of many domestic animals; transmitted in meat and milk; grow at refrigerator temperatures of 4°C; produce **endotoxins**
  - o Symptoms: diarrhea, fever, headache, abdominal pain; diagnosis: culture organism, serological tests; treatment: antibiotics, oral rehydration

- ● *Clostridium Perfringens* **Gastroenteritis**
  - o Form of food poisoning caused by gram positive (+), **obligately anaerobic endospore-forming rod** *Clostridium* perfringens; also causes human gas gangrene; associated with meats containing intestinal animal contents during slaughter; endospore survives most routine heating; grows in intestinal tract; produces **exotoxin;** symptoms: abdominal cramping and diarrhea; most cases mild and self-limiting; treatment: oral rehydration; diagnosis: isolate and identify pathogen in stool samples

- ● *Clostridium Difficile*-**Associated Diarrhea**
  - o Caused by gram positive (+), **endospore forming anaerobe** *Clostridium difficile* which produces **exotoxins;** in stool of many healthy individuals; symptoms: mild diarrhea to colitis (inflammation of the colon); colitis can result in ulceration, perforation of intestinal wall
  - o Disease precipitated by **extended use of antibiotics;** leads to elimination of most competing intestinal bacteria and rapid growth of the **toxin producing** *Clostridium difficile*; mostly in hospitals, nursing homes, day care centers; newer strain, **NAP1/BI/027,** can produce more **exotoxin** and occurring at near-epidemic rates; diagnosis: by immunoassay (detects responsible **exotoxins**), cytotoxin assay; treatment: discontinuation of antibiotics, oral hydration, metronidazole, fidaxomicin, vancomycin; for recurrences: rafiximin or nitazoxanide; enemas (of human stool)

- ***Bacillus cereus* Gastroenteritis**
  - o Caused by large, gram positive (+), **endospore-forming** bacterium *Bacillus cereus*; common in soil and vegetation; generally harmless; can cause foodborne illnesses; **spores** germinate as food cools after heating; grows rapidly and produces **toxins;** rice dishes, served in Asian restaurants susceptible; symptoms: diarrhea, nausea, vomiting; disease is self limiting; diagnosis: isolation of microbe from foods

E. Viral Diseases of the Digestive System

- **Mumps**
  - o Targets the **parotid glands**; begins with painful swelling of one or both glands; virus transmitted in saliva and respiratory secretions; portal of entry is respiratory tract; virus multiples in respiratory tract and lymph nodes in the neck; reach salivary glands via blood; **viremia occurs**; symptoms: inflammation and painful swelling of **parotids**, fever, pain during swallowing; can cause **orchitis** (inflammation of the testes) which could cause sterility; **meningitis**; inflammation of ovaries, pancreatitis; treatment: attenuated live vaccine administered as part of the trivalent measles, mumps, rubella **(MMR) vaccine**; diagnosis: symptoms, embryonated egg or cell culture, ELISA tests
- **Hepatitis**
  - o Inflammation of the liver, caused by at least **five different viruses;** can result from other viruses (**EBV, CMV**); drugs and chemical toxicity can also cause acute hepatitis
    - **Hepatitis A:** caused by *Hepatitis A virus* (HAV), Picornaviridae; **ssRNA, lacks envelope**; mode of transmission: oral/fecal; spreads: liver, kidney, spleen; shed in feces, detected in blood and urine; resistant to chlorine disinfectants; symptoms: anorexia, malaise, nausea, diarrhea, abdominal pain, fever chills; incubation: 2 to 6 weeks; diagnosis: detect IgM anti-HAV; treatment: immune globulin, inactivated vaccines (part of childhood vaccination schedule); high risk groups: homosexual men, IV drug users
    - **Hepatitis B:** caused by *Hepatitis B virus* (HBV), Hepadnaviridae; **dsDNA, has envelope**; transmission: parenteral, IV, sexual contact; present in body fluids: saliva, breast milk, semen; **serum** positive for HBV contains three distinct particles: **(1) Dane particle:** largest; **complete virion**; infectious and able to replicate, **(2) Spherical particles (SP):** smaller; unassembled component of the virion without nucleic acids, and **(3)Filamentous particles (FP):** tubular; unassembled component of the virion without nucleic acids; **SP** and **FP** contain **hepatitis B surface antigen (HBsAg)**, which can be detected using antibodies to them; used in screening of blood; high risk groups include: health care workers, IV drug user, persons undergoing hemodialysis; diagnosis: symptoms, liver function test; serologic tests (detect **HBV antigens and antibodies**): HBsAg-presence indicates virus in the blood; **HBeAg (**marker for **core of the virus)-virus is replicating vigorously;** prevention: disposable needles and syringes, barrier-type contraception, screening transfused blood, **HBV vaccines;** able to cultivate in cell culture; treatment: no specific treatment, antivirals: α-interferon, nucleoside analogues (lamivudine, adefovir, entecavir, telbivudine, tenofovir DF), liver transplants
      - ✓ Infection can be **acute or chronic**
        - ❖ **Acute Hepatitis B:** many cases person unaware; some patients suffer from low grade fever, nausea, vomiting, abdominal pain; jaundice, dark urine, liver damage may appear; long period of recovery persues; few cases develop into **fulminant hepatitis** (sudden massive liver damage)
        - ❖ **Chronic Hepatitis B:** hepatitis persists for more than **6 months;** for some the condition is asymptomatic; others may suffer from malaise, poor appetite, general fatigue; some results in liver cirrhosis, liver cancer

- **Hepatitis C:** caused by *Hepatitis C virus* (HCV), Flaviviridae; **ssRNA, has envelope**; form of transfusion-transmitted hepatitis; transmission: parenteral, IV drug users; doesn't kill infected cell, causes immune inflammatory response which clears infection or destroys liver; delay of 70-80 days between infection and detectable antibodies; considered a silent epidemic; detected during routine testing; symptoms: similar to Hepatitis B, can progress to chronic stage leading to cirrhosis or cancer; common cause for liver transplants; diagnosis: PCR; treatment: peginterferon and ribavirin combination
            - **Hepatitis D (Delta Hepatitis):** caused by *Hepatitis D virus* (HDV), Deltaviridae; **ssRNA;** develops **envelope** when external envelop **of HBsAg** covers **HDV protein core**; can propagate only in the **presense of HBV**; transmission: parenteral **coinfection with HBV**; can occur as acute **(coinfection form:** self limiting) or chronic **(superinfection form:** progressive liver damage and possible death) hepatitis; diagnosis: IgM antibodies; treatment: none, HBV vaccine protective
            - **Hepatitis E:** caused by *Hepatitis E virus* (HEV), Caliciviridae; **ssRNA, no envelope;** transmission: ingestion/fecal-oral; symptoms: clinically similar to HAV, high mortality in pregnant women; does not cause chronic liver disease; treatment: none, HAV vaccine protective
            - **Other Types of Hepatitis: Hepatitis F (HFV)** and **Hepatitis G (HGV);** both blood transmitted viruses
- **Viral Gastroenteritis**
    - Acute gastroenteritis one of the most common diseases of humans
        - **Rotovirus: dsRNA**; most common cause especially in infants and children; transmission: fecal/oral; symptoms: low grade fever, diarrhea, vomiting; shed in stool; diagnosis: enzyme immunoassays; treatment: oral rehydration, oral vaccine
        - **Norovirus: ssRNA;** transmission: fecal/oral from food, water, aerosols from vomitus; virus persistent on surfaces; symptoms: vomiting and/or diarrhea; effective measures to control: mechanical removal/hand washing, hypochlorite (bleach), peroxygen; diagnosis: PCR and EIA tests of stool; treatment: oral or IV rehydration

F. Fungal Diseases of the Digestive System
- Some fungi produce **mycotoxins** which cause disease
- Diagnosis based on finding fungi or **mycotoxins** in food
- **Ergot Poisoning**
    - *Claviceps purpurea* produces **mycotoxins**
    - *Claviceps purpurea* produce **smut** infections on grain crops
    - The **mycotoxins** cause **ergot poisoning (**or **ergotism)** resulting from eating rye or other cereals contaminated with the fungus; can result in gangrene, hallucinogenic symptoms like LSD
- **Aflatoxin Poisoning**
    - *Aspergillus flavus* produces the **mycotoxin aflatoxin**
    - **Aflatoxin** found in many foods but particularly on peanuts
    - Causes serious damage to livestock; in humans may contribute to cirrhosis and cancer of the liver

G. Protozoan Diseases of the Digestive System
- Several pathogenic protozoa complete their life cycle in humans digestive tract
- Usually ingested as resistant infective cysts
- **Giardiasis**
    - Caused by *Giardia lamblia* (also known as *Giardia intestinalis* and *Giardia duodenalis*); a flagellated protozoan which attaches to human intestinal wall; causes prolonged diarrhea, nausea, flatulence, weight loss, abdominal cramp

- o **Hydrogen sulfide odor** detected in breath or stools; cysts shed in feces; also shed by beavers
- o Transmitted by contaminated water supplies; cyst stage relatively insensitive to chlorine
- o Filtration, boiling necessary to eliminate cysts
- o Diagnosed: "**string test**", ELISA, fluorescent antibody **(FA)** test
- o Treatment: metronidazole, quinacrine hydrochloride, nitazoxanide
- **Cryptosporidiosis**
  - o Caused by *Cryptosporidium*; most prevalent species affecting humans are *Cryptosporidium parvum* and *Cryptosporidium hominis*; infection occurs when oocysts ingested; oocysts release sporozoites into small intestine; sporozoites invade wall; undergo a cycle releasing oocysts which are excreted in feces
  - o Transmission: contaminated recreational and drinking water systems via animal feces; contaminated lakes, streams, wells
  - o Causes diarrhea
  - o Relatively insensitive to chlorine; elimination of cysts by: filtration, ultraviolet radiation, ozonation, chlorine dioxide; diagnosis: AF stain, ELISA, FA tests
  - o Treatment: nitazoxanide, oral rehydration
- *Cyclospora* **Diarrheal Infection**
  - o Caused by *Cyclospora cayetanensis*; causes watery diarrhea; transmission: oocytes in contaminated water, on contaminated berries, uncooked food
  - o Diagnosed: oocysts by microscopic examination; treatment: combination of trimethoprim and sulfamethoxazole
- **Amoebic Dysentery (Amoebiasis)**
  - o Caused by *Entamoeba histolytica* transmitted in food or contaminated water by cysts; in intestine, cyst wall digested away and trophozoites released; multiply in epithelial cells in large intestine; causes a severe dysentery
  - o Abscess formation can occur; treated surgically if involving bowel, liver, other organs
  - o Diagnosed: microscopy, serology; treatment: metronidazole, surgery

H. Helminthic Diseases of the Digestive System
- Very common, especially in conditions of poor sanitation
- **Tapeworms**
  - o Life cycle: adult worm lives in intestine of human host; **produces eggs** which are excreted in the feces; eggs ingested by animals (cattle) and hatch into **larval** form called a **cysticerus** which lodges in animal's muscles; human infection due to eating undercooked beef, pork, fish containing **cysticerci**; cysticerci develop into **adult tapeworms** which attach to intestinal wall by **suckers on the scolex**
    - ■ *Taenia saginata* (**beef tapeworm**): causes vague abdominal discomfort
    - ■ *Taenia solium* (**pork tapeworm**): may produce **larva stage** in humans
    - ■ *Taenia asiatica* (**Asian tapeworm**): only in Asia
  - o **Taeniasis: adult tapeworm** infects human intestine; generally benign; eggs continuously expelled
  - o **Cysticercosis:** infection caused by the **larva stage** *Taenia solium*; humans or swine ingest *Taenia solium* eggs; **eggs** leave digestive tract and **develop into larvae** in tissue (muscle, eye, brain)
    - ■ Muscle tissue: relatively benign; few serious symptoms
    - ■ Eye: **ophthalmic cysticercosis**; affects vision
    - ■ Central nervous system: **neurocysticercosis**; symptoms mimic epilepsy or brain tumor
  - o *Diphyllobothrium latum* (**fish tapeworm**): found in trout, pike, perch, salmon; transmitted by eating raw fish (sushi, sashimi)
  - o Diagnosis of **tapeworms**: identify tapeworm eggs or segments (**proglottids**) in feces
  - o Treatment: praziquantel, albendazole

- **Hydatid Disease**
  - o Caused by **tapeworm** *Echinococcus granulosus*
  - o Adult form resides in intestinal tract of carnivorous animals (dogs, wolves)
  - o Humans infected from feces of the infected animal (example: dog which ate flesh of sheep containing cyst form of tapeworm)
  - o More common in persons raising sheep or hunt and trap wild animals; once ingested by humans, eggs migrates to tissues in the body (lungs, liver, brain); once in place, egg develops into a **hydatid cyst,** which grows; damage due to size and location; **cyst** can rupture producing daughter **cysts**
  - o **Cyst fluid** contains proteinaceous material which can result in anaphylactic shock
  - o Diagnosis: X-ray, CT, MRI; serological test
  - o Treatment: surgery, albendazole
- **Nematodes**
  - o **Pinworms:** disease caused by *Enterobius vermicularis*; migrates outside anus of human host to lay eggs, causing itching around anus; diagnosis: finding eggs around anus (**"scotch tape"** test); treatment: pyrantel pamoate, mebendazole
  - o **Hookworms:** most often seen in United States is *Necator americanus*; **larvae enter skin** from soil; attaches to intestinal wall; feeds on blood and tissue; symptoms: can lead to anemia, pica; diagnosed by microscopy (finding eggs in feces); treatment: mebendazole
    - ■ *Ancyclostoma duodenale*: another Hookworm distributed around the world
  - o **Ascariasis:** caused by *Ascaris lumbricoides*; common in southeastern United States; high incidence in children; diagnosis: adult worm emerges from mouth, anus, or nose; live on partially digested food in intestinal tract; life cycle: eggs shed in person's feces are ingested by another person; eggs hatch (in upper intestine) into larvae; larvae pass into bloodstream, then into lungs; migrate into throat and are swallowed; larvae develop into egg-laying adults in the intestines; can cause pulmonary symptoms; intestinal, bile duct, or pancreatic duct blockage; diagnosis: microscopy for eggs; treatment: mebendazole, albendazole
  - o **Whipworm: trichuriasis** caused by *Trichuris trichiura*: wide spread in the tropics; main body thin and hairlike, posterior end resembles a **coiled whip;** microscopy reveals **whipworm's distinctive egg shape** (tea tray with handles); eggs picked up by children in contaminated soil; egg ingested; hatches and enters intestinal glands; grows and tunnels back to interior intestinal surface; positions itself; feed on cell contents and blood: symptoms: anemia, malnutrition, weight loss, retarded growth; treatment: mebendazole, albendazole
  - o **Trichinellosis:** caused by *Trichinella spiralis*; ingested by eating uncooked pig, or eating flesh of animals that feed on **garbage** (bears); humans ingest flesh of infected animal; digestive action in intestine removes **cyst wall;** matures into adult form; adult produce **larvae; encysted larvae** lodge in human striated muscle; any ground meat can be contaminated from machinery used in grinding contaminated meats; symptoms: fever, swelling around eyes; freezing kills *Trichinella spiralis,* but not other species (*Trichinella native*); diagnosed: biopsy, serological tests, ELISA; treatment: mebendazole, albendazole, corticosteroids

MICROBIOLOGY

MICROBIAL DISEASES OF THE CARDIOVASCULAR AND LYMPHATIC SYSTEMS

A. Structure and Function of the Cardiovascular (CV) and Lymphatic Systems

- Cardiovascular System: to pump blood through the body's tissues; to deliver and remove substances from cells; consist of: heart, blood vessels, blood (formed elements and plasma)
- Lymphatic System consist of: lymph, lymph vessels, lymph nodes, lymphoid organs
  - o Some blood plasma may leak into spaces surrounding tissue cells (plasma now called interstitial fluid); enter lymph capillaries (now fluid called lymph); this lymph transported to larger vessels called lymphatics (contain valves); eventually all lymph will return to the blood, before the blood enters the heart (note: lymph must pass through lymphoid follicles (or nodules), lymph nodes, lymphoid organs)

B. Bacterial Diseases of the CV and Lymphatic Systems

- **Sepsis and Septic Shock**
  - o **Sepsis:** a systemic inflammatory response syndrome caused by a focus of infection that releases mediators of inflammation into the blood stream; fever, chills, rapid heart and respiratory rates, elevated white blood cell count
  - o **Septicemia:** illness associated with the persistent presence of pathogenic microbes or their toxins in the blood
  - o **Septic shock:** sepsis resulting in **drop in BP** and **dysfunction of organs**
  - o **Lymphangitis:** inflammation of the lymphatic vessels
  - o **Gram Negative (-) Sepsis:** cell wall (**LPS**) contains **endotoxins**; when released can cause drop in blood pressure; treatment: tricky (may aggravate conditions), neutralize **LPS** component and inflammatory cytokines, **drotrecogin alfa (Xigris)** approved
  - o **Gram Positive (+) Sepsis: now** most common cause of sepsis; produce **exotoxins**; caused mainly by invasive procedures; **enterococci:** *Enterococcus faecium* and *Enterococcus faecalis* are both leading cause of nosocomial infections; 90% now resistant to vancomycin; *Streptococcus agalactiae:* only and most common cause of **neonatal sepsis**
  - o **Puerperal Sepsis:** nosocomial infection; **an infection of the uterus** (childbirth or abortion) **and breast**; *Streptococcus pyogenes* (a group A β-hemolytic streptococcus) most common cause of the infection; can progress to: peritonitis, sepsis; treatment: penicillin
- **Bacterial Infections of the Heart**
  - o **Endocarditis:** inflammation of the endocardium (inner layer)
    - **Subacute bacterial endocarditis:** caused by α-hemolytic streptococci; enterococci or staphylococci are causes; microbes released by tooth extraction, tonsillectomy, body piercing; persons with abnormal heart valves cause bacteria to lodge in preexisting lesions; bacteria clump and become entrapped in blood clots; clots can break off and block vessels and affect circulation; in time heart valve becomes impaired
    - **Acute bacterial endocarditis:** more rapid progression; usually caused by *Staphylococcus aureus*
  - o **Pericarditis:** inflammation of the sac surrounding the heart (pericardium); can be caused by streptococci
  - o **Rheumatic Fever:** caused by *Streptococcus pyogenes*, considered an autoimmune complication; affects persons 3 to 18 years of age; follows an episode of streptococcal sore throat→arthritis,

163

fever; subcutaneous nodules; inflammation of the heart and heart valves →death; can develop into Sydenham's chorea (purposeless, involuntary movements during walking); treated with penicillin

o **Tularemia:** a zoonotic disease (disease transmitted by contact with infected animal); caused by *Francisella tularensis*: gram-negative pleomorphic rod-shaped bacteria; facultative anaerobe; vector usually small wild animals (rabbits), insects; enter humans at abrasion site, eating undercooked meat, or bitten by diseased animal; survive in body due to inability to be phagocytized; produce ulcers→ lymphangitis→ septicemia→ pneumonia→death; concern use for biological warfare; treatment: tetracycline

o **Brucellosis (Undulant Fever):** world's most common bacterial zoonosis; small gram-negative aerobic coccoid rods; easily airborne; possible agent of bioterrorism; multiply in the uterus of infected animals; symptoms in humans include: fever, chills, malaise→night sweats and fever→death; treatment: combination of at least two antibiotics; three species of importance:

- *Brucella arbortus*: in cattle, camels, bison
- *Brucella suis*: mostly swine; also in cattle
- *Brucella melitensis*: most serious pathogen; goats and sheep; excreted in unpasteurized food products

o **Anthrax:** caused by *Bacillus anthracis*; gram positive (+) aerobic endospore forming microbe; grows well in soil; concern as an agent of bioterrorism; strikes grazing animals (cattle, sheep); humans infected by handling infected animals, hide, wool; handling leads to pustules→septicemia; primary virulent factor are two **exotoxins** (edema toxin and lethal toxin) which share **a third toxin component** (cell receptor binding protein called protective antigen); livestock vaccinated as a precaution; treatment: ciprofloxacin or doxycycline plus one or more additional agents, raxibacumab; vaccine approved for humans; **Anthrax affects humans in three forms:**

- **Cutaneous:** contact with material containing endospores; papule develops→vesicles→depressed ulcerated area covered by a **black eschar (scab)** around point of infection
- **Gastrointestinal:** ingestion of undercooked food; n/v/abdominal pain; ulceration in GI tract
- **Inhalational** (pulmonary): most dangerous form; endospores inhaled→pneumonia; **Woolsorter's disease:** inhaled endospores→ pneumonia

o **Gangrene:** the result of soft tissue death due to **ischemia; ischemia:** loss/interruption of blood supply; **ischemia** can lead to **necrosis** (death of the tissue); substances released from **necrotic** tissue provide nutrients for certain bacteria; species of *Clostridium* grow well in such conditions; *Clostridium*: gram positive (+), rod shaped, endospore forming anaerobes; found in soil, intestinal tract of humans and domesticated animals

- *Clostridium perfringens*: most commonly involved in **gangrene;** grow and ferment carbohydrates in tissue→gases→tissue swells→systemic illness; seen in improperly performed abortions; treatment: debridement, surgical removal, amputation, **hyperbaric chamber,** penicillin

o **Systemic Diseases Caused by Bites and Scratches:** usually by animal bites (dogs, cats)

- **Animal Bites:** *Pasteurella multocida*: gram negative (-) rod; pathogen of animals; can cause pneumonia and septicemia; treatment: penicillin and tetracycline
- **Cat-Scratch Disease:** caused by *Bartonella henselae*: an aerobic, gram negative (-) bacterium; primarily transmitted by scratch →swelling lymph node; usually self-limited (resolves on its own)
- **Rat-Bite Fever:** caused by rats; common in large urban areas; affects children and adults; two similar but distinct diseases (both treated with penicillin or doxycycline) are:
    - ✓ Streptobacillary rat-bite fever: caused by *Streptobacillus moniliformis*

     ✓ Spirillar fever: known as sodoku (Asia); caused by *Spirillum minus*
- o   **Vector-Transmitted Diseases**
  - ■ **Plague** (also known as **Black Death**): caused by gram negative (-) rod *Yersinia pestis*; transmitted from one rat to another by rat flea (*Xenopsylla cheopis*); organism enters blood stream and multiples in lymph nodes; in groin and armpit, node enlarges **(buboes)** →fever→death; **septicemic plague** the organism causes septic shock; carried to lungs causing disease called **pneumonic plague;** treatment: streptomycin and tetracycline; vaccine is available
  - ■ **Relapsing Fever:** caused by all members of spirochete genus *Borrelia* (except for the species causing Lyme Disease); transmitted by ticks which feed on rodents; disease characterized by: fever, jaundice, rose colored skin spots; fever subsides; relapse; treatment: tetracycline
  - ■ **Lyme Disease (Lyme Borreliosis):** caused by spirochete *Borrelia burgdorferi*; transmitted by ticks (*Ixodes pacificus* and *Ixodes scapularis*); field mice most important reservoir; starts out as a rash at bite site→clears in the center as it expands (**bull's eye rash**)→ rash fades; flulike symptoms appear→ can lead to cardiac and neurological symptoms; later can develop arthritis; diagnosis difficult; treatment: antibiotics
  - ■ **Ehrlichiosis and Anaplasmosis:** symptoms of both same (flulike symptoms: high fever, headache); treatment same: doxycycline
    - ✓ **Human monocytotropic ehrlichiosis (HME):** caused by *Ehrlichiosis chafeenis*: gram negative (-) rickettsia-like, obligately intracellular bacterium; morulae form within cytoplasm of monocytes; vector is the Lone star tick
    - ✓ **Human granulocytic anaplasmosis (HGA);** formerly called **humans granulocytic ehrlichiosis;** caused by *Anaplasma phagocytophilum*; an obligate intracellular bacterium; morulae formation also; tick vector is *Ixodes scapularis*
  - ■ **Typhus Diseases:** caused by rickettsias (intracellular obligate parasites); rickettsias spread by arthropods; infect mostly endothelial cells of the vascular system; the inflammation leads to blockage, rupture of small blood vessels
    - ✓ **Epidemic Typhus:** caused by *Rickettsia prowazekii*; carried by human body louse *Pediculus humanus corporis*; transmitted when feces of louse enters skin; spreads in crowded unsanitary conditions (Anne Frank); symptoms: fever→stupor, rash of small red spots→ death; treatment: tetracycline and chloramphenicol effective; vaccines available
    - ✓ **Endemic Murine Typhus:** caused by *Rickettsia typhi*; transmitted from rodents to humans by rat flea *Xenopsylla cheopis*. Treatment: tetracycline and chloramphenicol effective
    - ✓ **Spotted Fevers**
      - ❖ **Rocky Mountain Spotted fever:** caused by *Rickettsia rickettsii*; parasite of ticks; passed from one tick generation to the next by **transovarian passage;** different ticks involved: *Dermacentor andersoni* (wood tick), *Dermacentor variabilis* (dog tick); symptoms: tick bite→ macular rash (on palms and soles) with fever and headache→stupor→death; treatment: chloramphenicol and tetracycline effective

D. Viral Diseases of the CV and Lymphatic Systems
- ● **Burkitts's Lymphoma**
  - o   Most common childhood cancer in Africa; fast growing affecting the jaw
  - o   Caused by a herpes-like virus named *Epstein-Barr virus* (**EBV**)
  - o   Official name is *human herpesvirus 4* (**HHV-4**)
  - o   **EBV** associated with **Burkitt's Lymphoma**
  - o   In the United States, **Burkitts's Lymphoma rare**, and usually abdominal

- **Infectious Mononucleoisis**
  - o Caused by **EBV**: multiplies in parotid glands; route of infection by transfer of saliva (kissing, sharing drinking vessels)
  - o Resting memory B cells, in lymphoid tissue, primary site of replication
  - o Lymphocytes have unusual lobed nuclei in blood during acute infection
  - o Symptoms: fever, swollen lymph nodes involving neck, sore throat, due to responses of T cells to infection
  - o Infected B cells produce **heterophile antibodies** (weak antibodies) used in diagnosis
  - o Self-limiting; can lead to ruptured spleen
- **Epstein-Barr Virus and other Diseases**
  - o Diseases associated with **EBV**, but not proven: Multiple sclerosis, Hodgkin's disease, Nasopharyngeal cancer
- **Cytomegalovirus (CMV) Infections**
  - o Large herpes-virus; official name is **human herpesvirus 5 (HHV-5)**; may remain latent in white blood cells; shed in body secretions (saliva, semen, breast mild); transmission: kissing, sexual, blood transfusions, transplanted tissue, day care centers; forms inclusion bodies (bodies in pairs called **"owl's eyes"**) in infected cells; infected cells enlarge, also; disease of newborns named **cytomegalic inclusion disease (CID)** with symptoms including severe mental retardation and/or hearing loss; in healthy adults infection causes no symptoms or mild mononucleosis; **CMV** opportunistic pathogen for immunocompromised individuals (causes pneumonia, **CMV retinitis**); treatment: immunoglobulin preparations, ganciclovir, cidofovir
- **Chikungunya Fever**
  - o Tropical disease caused by *Alphavirus Chikungunya virus*; symptoms: high fever, severe crippling joint pain, rash, blisters; vectors are mosquitoes: *Aedes aegypti* and *Aedes albopictus*
- **Classic Viral Hemorrhagic Fevers**
  - o Most are zoonotic diseases
    - ■ **Yellow Fever:** caused by *Flavivirus Yellow fever virus*; endemic; monkeys are natural reservoir; injected into skin by mosquito *Andes aegypti*; symptoms: fever, chills, headaches, n/v→jaundice→possible death; treatment: none, there is a vaccine
    - ■ **Dengue:** caused by *Flavivirus Dengue virus*; causes milder disease (**dengue fever,** also known as **breakbone fever**) and is rarely fatal; transmitted by *Andes aegypti* (human to human); symptoms: fever, severe muscle and joint pain, rash; a severe form, **dengue hemorrhagic fever (DHF)** can cause shock, and kill within hours
- **Emerging Viral Hemorraghic Fevers**
  - o Considered new or emerging viruses
    - ■ **Marburg virus** or **green monkey virus:** shaped in the form of a filament (filoviruses); from imported African monkeys; symptoms: headache, muscle pain; high fever vomiting blood and bleeding internally and externally
    - ■ **Ebola hemorrhagic fever:** caused by *Ebola virus* : a filovirus similar to **Marburg virus;** damages walls to blood vessels and interferes with coagulation; natural host reservoir is fruit bat; unsterilized needles; person to person
    - ■ **Lassa fever:** caused by an *Arenavirus*, the *Lassa virus*; rodent reservoir; person to person body fluids
    - ■ **Argentine** and **Bolivian hemorrhagic fevers:** transmitted by contact with rodent excretions
    - ■ **Whitewater Arroyo virus:** reservoir in wood rats
    - ■ *Hantavirus* **pulmonary syndrome (HPS):** caused by *Sin Nombre virus* (a Bunyarvirus); fatal pulmonary infection (lungs fill with fluid); antiviral ribavirin recommended; in Asia and Europe, known as **hemorrhagic fever with renal syndrome** (primarily affects renal function)

E. Protozoan Diseases of the CV and Lymphatic Systems
- Those causing diseases often have complex life cycles
- **American Trypanosomiasis (Chagas' Disease)**
  - Involves the cardiovascular system; caused by *Trypanosoma cruzi*; flagellated; reservoir include: rodents, armadillos, opossums: vector is the reduviid bug (also called kissing bug); acute stage: fever, swollen glands; chronic stage: **megaesophagus and megacolon**, congenital infections; treatment: nifurtimox and benznidazole
- **Toxoplasmosis**
  - Involves cardiovascular and lymphatic systems; caused by *Toxoplasma gondii* (spore forming protozoan); cats main reservoir; undergoes sexual phase in intestinal tract of cats; immature oocytes shed in feces; mature oocytes ingested by other animals via contaminated water or food→ can lead to tissue cyst which can persist in the brain; **congenital infection in fetus**→stillbirth or brain and/or visual damage; treatment: if pregnant woman positive (by serological test) abortion encouraged, treated with pyrimethamine in combination with sulfadiazine and folinic acid
- **Malaria**
  - Caused by parasite *Plasmodium*; mosquito vector *Anopheles*; also transmitted by unsterilized syringes, blood transfusions; symptoms: fever, chills, vomiting, headache, at 2 to 3 day intervals, alternating with asymptomatic periods
  - Four major forms of malaria
    - *Plasmodium vivax*: most prevalent form; considered benign; can remain dormant in liver
    - *Plasmodium ovale*: relatively benign malaria; lower in incidence; restricted geographically
    - *Plasmodium malariae*: same as *Plasmodium ovale*
    - *Plasmocium falciparum*: **most dangerous; malignant malaria;** infects more red blood cells than other forms; can lead to tissue death (kidney, liver); cause of cerebral malaria
  - Disease and symptoms related to complex reproductive cycle: infection started by bite of mosquito (carries sporozoites in saliva)→blood→sporozoites enter liver→ in liver undergo reproductive schizogony→ results in release of merozoites into blood stream→ merozoites infect red blood cells→again merzoite undergoes schizogony→red blood cells lyse and new merozoites released; new merozoites infect red blood cells to renew the cycle; some merozoites develop into male and female gametocytes→ enter digestive tract of mosquito→ go through a sexual cycle which produces infective sporozoites
  - Vaccines: **transmission-blocking vaccine:** antibodies produced by human host to be delivered to the biting mosquito; diagnosis by blood smear; antigen detecting test; prophylxis (chloroquine, combination of atovaquone and proquanil); therapy (chloroquine, malarone or oral quinine); worldwide treatment: artemisinin combination therapies (**ACT**); prevention: combination of vector control, chemotherapeutics, immunological approaches
- **Leishmaniasis**
  - Transmitted by female sandfly
  - Infective form (**promastigote**) in saliva of the insect; loses its flagellum (becomes an **amastigote**) which proliferates in phagocytic cells; **amastigote** ingested by feeding sandflies, which renews the cycle; infection in humans caused by: insect bite, contact with contaminated blood (transfusion, shared needles)
  - Classified into three groups
    - *Leishmania donovani* (**Visceral Leishmaniasis**): known as **kala azar** in India; parasite invades internal organs; symptoms: chills, fever, sweating; invade and proliferate in the liver, spleen, kidneys→death. Treatment: sodium stilbogluconate, liposomal amphotericin B, paromomycin
    - *Leishmania tropica* (**Cutaneous Leishmaniasis**): cause skin lesions sometimes called **oriental sore**; papule at bite site→ulceration→ scar

- *Leishmania braziliensis* (**Mucocutaneous Leishmaniasis**): also known as **American leishmaniasis;** cause skin and mucous membrane lesions; disfigures mouth, nose, throat
- **Babesiosis**
  - Disease in United States caused by *Babesia microti*; transmitted by tick; replicate in red blood cells→anemia; disease resembles malaria; symptoms: fever, chills, night sweats; serious in immunocompromised patients; treatment: atovarquone, azithromycin

F. Helminthic Diseases of the CV and Lymphatic Systems

- The Cardiovascular System is used for the life cycle of many helminthes
- **Schistosomiasis**
  - Disease caused by **a fluke**; symptoms results from eggs shed by adult schistosomes in human host
  - Adult consist of a female living inside groove of a male; union between the two produce new eggs; some of the eggs end up in tissue; leads to formation of **granulomas;** some eggs excreted and enter water cycle
  - Disease spread by human feces or urine carrying eggs of the schistosome (enter water supply) →eggs hatch free swimming larvae (**miracidia**)→infect snail→**miracidium** reproduce producing **cercariae**→ **cercariae** released from snail→penetrate skin of human; travel through circulatory system to blood vessels in intestine→mature into adults
  - Symptoms: local granulomas; liver, brain, and lung damage
  - Three groups
    - *Schistosoma haematobium*: causes inflammation of the urinary bladder wall; Africa, Middle East
    - *Schistosoma japonicum*: inflammation of the liver, spleen, intestinal; east Asia
    - *Schistosoma mansoni*: inflammation of the liver, LI; South America, Caribbean, Puerto Rico
  - Treatment: praziquantel, oxamniquine
- **Swimmer's Itch**
  - Caused by a fluke; common in lakes in Northern United States; mature in wildfowl and not in humans
  - Cutaneous **allergic reaction to cercariae**, similar to **schistosomiasis**

MICROBIOLOGY

ENVIRONMENTAL MICROBIOLOGY

A. Metabolic Diversity and Habitats
- Microbes are essential in the maintenance of life
- They live in widely varied habitats (hot springs, Antarctic regions, under rocks)
- **Extremophiles:** microbes which are able to live in extreme conditions of temperature, alkalinity, acidity, or salinity
  - The enzymes, **extremozymes**, makes growth under these conditions, tolerable
    - Example: *Thermus aquaticus* (grows in hot springs; heat-resistant *Taq polymerase* enzyme)
  - In their environment, microorganisms must be able to compete with other microbes for nutrients; they may metabolize common nutrients at a faster rate or use nutrients that competing microbes cannot metabolize
    - Example: **Lactic acid bacteria** (not able to use oxygen as an electron acceptor; ferments sugars to lactic acid (acid), leaving most of energy unused); this acidity inhibits growth of competing microbes
- **Symbiosis**
  - The interaction between coexisting populations or organisms
  - Most important economical example of an **animal-microbe symbiosis: ruminants** (have a digestive organ called a **rumen**); Example: sheep, cattle; graze on cellulose rich plants; bacteria in rumen ferment cellulose into compounds which are eventually used for carbon and energy
  - **Mycorrhizae** (fungi): two primary types (**endomycorrhizae** and **ectomycorrhizae**); both extent surface area of plants roots to absorb nutrients; Example: *Truffles*

B. Soil Microbiology and Biogeochemical Cycles
- Most numerous organisms in soil are bacteria (millions of bacteria/gram)
- Microbial population of soil largest in top few centimeters; declines with depth
- **Soil** considered a **"biological fire"**; falling leaf is consumed by this **"fire"** as microbes in soil metabolize leafs organic matter; elements in leaf enter the **biogeochemical cycles** for: carbon, nitrogen, and sulfur
- In **biogeochemical cycles**: elements are oxidized and reduced by microbes to meet their metabolic needs
- **The Carbon Cycle**
  - The **primary biogeochemical cycle**
  - Plants, microbes, animals: **contain carbon in the form of organic compounds** (carbohydrates, fats, lipids, proteins)
  - **Steps**
    - First step of the carbon cycle is **photosynthesis**; **photoautotrophs** (cyanobacteria, green plants, algae, green and purple sulfur bacteria) **fix** (incorporate) carbon dioxide into organic matter using energy from the sun
    - Next step, **chemoheterotrophs** (animals, protozoa) eat **autotrophs**; the organic compounds of the **autotrophs** are digested, resynthesized; the carbon atoms of carbon dioxide are transferred from organism to organism up the food chain
    - **Chemoheterotrophs** use some of the organic molecules for their own energy needs; when this energy is released through **respiration**, carbon dioxide becomes available to start the cycle over again

- Much of the carbon remains within the organisms, until they excrete it or die; when plants or animals die, these organic compounds are decomposed (by bacteria, fungi); during decomposition, organic compounds are oxidized, and carbon dioxide is returned to the cycle
  - o Carbon is stored in rocks (lime stone) and is dissolved as carbonate ions in oceans
  - o Fossil organic material exist in the form of fossil fuels (coal, petroleum); burning fossil fuels release carbon dioxide (increase in atmosphere); possible cause of Global warming??
- **The Nitrogen Cycle**
  - o Nitrogen needed by all organisms for the synthesis of: proteins, nucleic acids, other nitrogen-containing compounds
  - o Nitrogen must be fixed (taken up and combined into organic compounds) for plants to use
  - o Specific microbes are important in the conversion of nitrogen to useable forms
  - o **Steps**
    - **Proteolysis:** organism dies; microbial decomposition results in the **breakdown of proteins into amino acids (aa's); aa's:** may be used by microbes for their own synthesis, absorbed by plants **(mycorrhizae), or deaminated to yield ammonia**

Proteinases   Peptidases
Proteins $\longrightarrow$ peptides/polypeptides $\longrightarrow$ **amino acids (aa's)**

Examples of microbes involved: *Pseudomonas, Bacillus*

- **Ammonification:** process which **aa's** are removed, degraded, and converted into ammonia
  - ✓ The **aa's** released undergo **deamination:** process in which the nitrogen containing amino group is removed; this process leads to production of ammonia, called **ammonification** (the release of ammonia); **ammonification** mediated by numerous bacteria and fungi

Microbial Ammonification
Amino acids (aa's) $\longrightarrow$ **Ammonia (NH_3)**

Examples of microbes involved: *Clostridium, Micrococcus, Proteus*

- **Nitrification:** step where **ammoniacal nitrogen/ammonia** is released and oxidized to **nitrates.** Soil which has: good aeration, rich in calcium carbonate, temperature below 30° C, neutral pH, less organic matter are favorable for **nitrification**
  - ✓ A **two stage process**, each performed by a **different group of bacteria**

Stage 1: **Ammonia** $\longrightarrow$ Nitrite ion (NO_2^-) (Example of microbe involved: *Nitrosomonas*)
Stage 2: Nitrite ion $\longrightarrow$ **Nitrate ion (NO_3^-)** (Example of microbe involved: *Nitrobacter*)

- **Denitrification: reverse process; loss of nitrogen** into the atmosphere; especially as nitrogen gas
  - ✓ Occurs in waterlogged soils (little oxygen available)

Nitrate ion$\rightarrow$ Nitrite ion$\rightarrow$Nitrous oxide $\rightarrow$**Nitrogen gas**

Example of microbes involved: *Pseudomonas, Bacillus*

- ■ **Nitrogen Fixation:** process in which **nitrogen gas** (in the atmosphere) is converted to **ammonia**; few species of bacteria, including cyanobacteria, can use nitrogen directly, as a nitrogen source; bacteria responsible for nitrogen fixation rely on **nitrogenase**, an enzyme
  - ✓ **Nitrogen fixation** is brought about by two types of microbes:
    - ❖ **Free-living Nitrogen-Fixing Bacteria:** found in high concentrations in the **rhizosphere** (a region from the plant root); region rich in nutrients in the soil
      - *Azotobacter, Beijerinckia*: **aerobic**
      - *Clostridium pasteurianum*: **anaerobic**
      - *Cyanobacteria*: **aerobic, photosynthesizing**; carry **nitrogenase** in **heterocysts**
  - ✓ **Nitrogen fixation** is brought about by two types of microbes **(Cont.)**
    - ❖ **Symbiotic Nitrogen-Fixing Bacteria:** certain bacteria infect the roots of **leguminous plants** (soybeans, peas, beans, peanuts, alfalfa, clover); they form **root nodules**; nitrogen then fixed by a symbiotic process of plant and bacteria; plant provides anaerobic environment and nutrients for the bacteria; bacteria fix nitrogen which can be incorporated into plant protein; examples: *Rhizobium, Bradyrhizobium*
      - **Nonleguminous plants**: alder trees; symbiotically infected with *Frankia* (an actinomycete) and forms a nitrogen fixing **root nodule**

Lichens: combination of fungus and an algae or a cyanobacterium

- ● **The Sulfur Cycle**
  - o Reduced forms of sulfur are **sulfides** (like the odorous gas hydrogen sulfide (H_2S)), and are energy sources for some microbes
  - o Sulfate-reducing bacteria grow in anaerobic environments; they reduce sulfur-containing amino acids to **hydrogen sulfide (H_2S)**; hydrogen sulfide **accumulates in anaerobic environments** (mud, swamps) giving of an odor of rotten eggs
  - o Photosynthetic bacteria metabolize the hydrogen sulfide anaerobically; they oxidize the H_2S, releasing sulfur as elemental sulfur; elemental sulfur accumulates in the soil
  - o Species of sulfur bacteria, including: *Thiobacillus, Beggiato, Thiothrix*; they also metabolize hydrogen sulfide, converting it to sulfate ions, which are then made available to plants for amino acid formation
  - o **Dissimilation:** proteins are decomposed and **sulfur is released as H_2S** to reenter the cycle
- ● **Life without Sunshine**
  - o Some biological communities can **exist without photosynthesis; they use the energy of H_2S**
  - o Such communities occur in deep sea vents; deep caves totally isolated from sunlight which support certain biological communities
  - o The **primary producers** in these communities: **chemoautotrophic bacteria**
  - o **Endoliths** (inside rocks) **are bacteria** which grow with little oxygen and nutrients; inside the rocks, chemical reactions and radioactivity split water, producing hydrogen, which can be used for energy by **autotrophic endolithic bacteria**; **carbon dioxide** serves as a carbon source; nutrients, especially nitrogen, very small
- ● **The Phosphorus Cycle**
  - o **Phosphorus** exist primarily as phosphate ions (PO_4^{3-}); **the phosphorus cycle** involves changes from soluble to insoluble forms, and from organic to inorganic phosphate depending on **pH**
    - ■ Example: *Thiobacillus*: produces acid
  - o In this cycle, **phosphorus** is not returned to the atmosphere; **accumulates in the seas**; retrieved via mining by man or seabirds
- ● **The Degradation of Synthetic Chemicals in Soil and Water**
  - o Many organic material (fallen leaves, animal residues) are readily degraded

- o Many chemicals which do not occur in nature, like plastics (called **xenobiotics**), enter the soil, and are not readily degraded by microbes
- o Solution: biodegradable plastics made from **polylactide (PLA)**, produced by lactic acid fermentation; another product is **polyhydroxyalkanoate (PHA)**
- o Many synthetic insecticides, example (**DDT**) are resistant to biodegradation
- o Some synthetic chemicals are made up of bonds/subunits which can be attacked by bacterial enzymes
  - Ex: **2,4-D** (kills lawn weed) and **2,4,5-T** (kills shrubs); both components of **Agent Orange**
- o Problems arise where toxic material, which are not biodegradable or degrade slowly, leach into ground waters→contamination→environmental and economic damage
- o **Bioremediation:** the use of microbes to degrade or detoxify pollutants
  - Example: Oil spills (petroleum) use bacteria and "fertilizer" containing nitrogen and phosphorus
  - **Bioaugmentation:** the addition of selected microbes (selected for growth, genetically modified)
- **The Degradation of Synthetic Chemicals in Soil and Water (Cont.)**
  - o **Solid Municipal Waste:** also known as garbage, placed in large compact landfills
    - Conditions: largely **anaerobic** and dry; can affect biodegradation of materials by microbes
    - Such **anaerobic** conditions promote the activity of **methanogens**, which produce **methane**
    - The **methane** can be used to generate energy
  - o **Composting:** process to convert plant remains into natural humus
    - Leaves or grass clippings will undergo microbial breakdown; **thermophilic bacteria**, under the right conditions, will raise the temperature of the compost in a few days; temperature will decline, and the pile can be turned, renewing the oxygen supply, and second temperature rise will occur; overtime, the **thermophilic microbes** will be replaced by **mesophilic population**, which continues the conversion into a stable material like humus

C. Aquatic Microbiology and Sewage Treatment

- **Aquatic Microbiology:** the study of microbes and their activities in **natural waters**
- Natural waters include: lakes, ponds, streams, rivers, estuaries, oceans
- Industrial and domestic **wastewater** enter lakes and stream, which affects aquatic life
- **Aquatic Microorganisms**
  - o Large numbers of microbes in a body of water usually indicate high nutrient levels in the water
  - o Contamination from sewage systems or biodegradable industrial organic wastes high in bacterial numbers
  - o In water with **low nutrient concentrations**, microbes tend to grow on **stationary surfaces** and **particulate matter**
  - o Many microbes, in which the habitat is water, often have appendages (Example: *Caulobacter*)
  - o **Freshwater Microbiota**
    - Freshwater microbial populations affected mainly by the availability of light and oxygen; photosynthetic algae are the main source of organic matter (energy)
    - Freshwater (lake, pond) has various zones and kinds of microbes found in each zone
      - ✓ **Littoral zone:** along the shore; rooted vegetation's; light penetrates throughout
      - ✓ **Limnetic zone:** surface of the open water area away from the shore; photosynthetic algae; Pseudomonads, *Caulobacter, Cytophaga, Hyphomicrobium*
      - ✓ **Profundal zone:** under limnetic zone; low oxygen and light levels; purple and green sulfur bacteria (both anaerobic, photosynthetic)
      - ✓ **Benthic zone:** contains sediment; low O_2 and light levels; *Desulfovibrio*, methane producing bacteria, *Clostridium species*

- o **Seawater Microbiota**
  - Bacteria, mostly **archaea**, located in seafloor sediments; make large amounts of methane gas
  - In sunlit water of the ocean, **photosynthetic cyanobacteria**, *Synchococcis* and *Prochloroccus* are abundant
  - Support of ocean life depends on photosynthetic **phytoplankton,** which are the basic ocean food chain; use energy from photosynthesis and atmospheric carbon dioxide for carbon; examples: *Trichodesmium* (cyanobacterium), *Pelagibacter ubique* (bacterium)
  - Many bacteria serve as food for larger consumers; first the protozoa, which are prey for planktonic animal life (krill); krill become prey for fish, and so on, up the food chain
  - Waters below 100 meters, planktonic members of **archaea genus** *Crenarchaeota,* make up most of the microbial biomass of the ocean; their carbon primarily from dissolved carbon dioxide
  - Deep-sea life is associated with **bioluminescence,** or light emission; consists of **bioluminescent** bacteria which have symbiotic relationships with **benthic-dwelling fish**; the **"light"** of these resident bacteria help attract and capture prey; the **bioluminescent** bacteria have an enzyme called **luciferase**, which emits the electron's energy as a photon of light
- ● **The Role of Microorganisms in Water Quality**
  - o Water in nature seldom totally pure
  - o **Water Pollution**
    - Form of primary interest due to microbial pathogenic organisms
  - o **Transmission of Infectious Diseases**
    - The most dangerous form of pollution due to feces entering the water; many diseases sustained by **fecal-oral route** of transmission
    - Examples: typhoid fever, cholera
  - o **Chemical Pollution**
    - Mainly from industrial and agricultural chemicals which have leached from the land, and enter the water in forms resistant to biodegradation
    - Rural waters have **excessive amounts of nitrate** (from agricultural fertilizers); when ingested by bacteria in gastrointestinal tract, converted to nitrite; excessive amounts compete for oxygen, which can be harmful to infants (**methemoglobinemia**)
    - Excessive amounts of **mercury**, from industrial water pollution, can be converted by bacteria into methyl mercury; taken up by fish; incorporated into human diet; **mercury** poisoning leading to serious **CNS** effects
    - Excessive amounts of chemicals also include: **pesticides, fluorides, synthetic detergents**
    - Biodegradable detergents, better, but contain **phosphates**; **abundance** of **phosphates** can lead to **eutrophication**
    - **Eutrophication: over nourishment,** due to pollutants or natural nutrients, of the aquatic ecosystems
    - **Red tides**, of toxin-producing phytoplankton, caused by excessive nutrients from oceanic upwelling's or terrestrial wastes
    - Coal-mining waste very high in **sulphur content**; bacteria such as *Thiobacillus ferrooxidins* converts the sulfur into sulfate; →sulfate enters stream as sulfuric acid
  - o **Water Purifying Tests**
    - Tests have been developed to determine the safely of water
    - Tests today aimed at detecting particular **indicator organisms**
    - Criteria for an **indicator organism:** the microbe is consistently present in human feces, in substantial numbers, so that its detection is a good indication that human waste is entering the water; it can be detected by simple tests
    - The usual **indicator organisms**, in the United States, are **coliform bacteria**

- ✓ **Coliform:** aerobic or facultative anaerobic, gram negative (-), non-endospore-forming, rod-shaped that ferment lactose to form gas within 48hrs at 35 °C, when placed in lactose broth; coliforms not pathogenic under normal conditions
- ✓ Many standards for food and water specify the identification of **fecal coliforms,** predominant one being *E. coli*
- ✓ **Methods** for determining **coliforms** in water, based largely on lactose-fermenting ability
    - ❖ The multiple-tube method: used to estimate the most probable number (**MPN**) method
    - ❖ The membrane filtration method: more direct
    - ❖ Media containing two substrates, **ONPG and MUG,** newer and more convenient method
      *****Coliforms:** produce β-galactosidase; acts on **ONPG**→yellow (+ presence)
      *****E.coli:** produces β-glucoronidase; acts on **MUG**→blue fluorescence (+ presence)
- ✓ **Coliforms** have limitations: some are indigenous
- Some pathogens (protozoan cyst, oocysts, viruses) more resistant to chemical disinfectants (chlorination) than **coliforms**
    - ✓ Examples: *Giardia lamblia* (cysts), *Cryptosporidium* (oocyst)
- **Water Treatment**
  - o Water obtained from uncontaminated reservoirs, fed by clear mountain streams or deep wells, requires minimal treatment in making it safe to drink
  - o Water, from polluted sources such as rivers which have received municipal and industrial wastes upstream, must undergo several steps in order to be purified of disease-causing microbes
  - o Steps involved in **Water Treatment**
    - **Coagulation and Filtration**
      - ✓ Turbid (raw/cloudy) water stands in a holding reservoir for a period of time; allows particulate matter to settle
      - ✓ Water then undergoes **flocculation:** where a chemical (such as alum) forms aggregates of suspended particles, called **flocs;** these **flocs** entrap colloidal material and carry it to the bottom
      - ✓ The water is then treated by **filtration** (through sand, anthracite coal, activated charcoal)
    - **Disinfection**
      - ✓ Before entering the municipal distribution system, filtered water disinfected by: **chlorination, ozone treatment, or exposed to UV light**
    - **Stored:** before use by consumer
- **Sewage (Wastewater) Treatment**
    - ✓ Includes all water from: washing, toilet waste, rain water running into street drains, some industrial waste
    - ✓ In the past, raw sewage (treated or untreated) was discharged into rivers or oceans
    - ✓ In the United States, most cases of discharge have been improved
    - ✓ Steps involved in **Sewage Treatment**
    - **Primary Sewage Treatment**
      - ✓ **Large floating materials in the wastewater are screened out; sewage is allowed to flow through chambers to remove sand and grit; skimmers remove oil and grease; floating debris is shredded and ground**
      - ✓ The **sewage** passes through sedimentation tanks; here more solid matter settles out; the **sewage solids** collecting on the bottom called **sludge;** at this stage, **called primary sludge**
      - ✓ The **sludge** is removed; the liquid flowing out (**effluent**) undergoes **secondary treatment**

- **Biochemical Oxygen Demand (BOD)**: measures the biologically degradable organic matter in water; **BOD:** is determined by the amount of oxygen the bacteria need to degrade the organic material; the **more oxygen used up as bacteria degrade organic matter in the sample, the greater the BOD**; Primary Sewage Treatment removes 25-35% of the **BOD**
- **Secondary Sewage Treatment**
  - ✓ Is predominantly **biological;** designed to **remove most of the organic material** and **reduce the BOD**
  - ✓ The **sewage** undergoes **aeration** (encourages growth of aerobic bacteria and microbes which oxidize the dissolved matter to carbon dioxide and water)
  - ✓ Two commonly used methods of **Secondary Treatment**: **Activated sludge system** and **Trickling filters**
    - ❖ **Activated sludge system:** in the aeration tanks, air or pure oxygen is passed through the effluent from **primary treatment**; some of the sludge from a previous batch is added to the incoming sewage; this **"inoculum"** contains large numbers of microbes efficient in degrading the sewage organic matter into carbon dioxide and water; one member of these microbes are *Zooglea* bacteria, which form masses in the aeration tanks called **sludge granules;** sometimes the sludge floats, rather than settles, **called bulking; bulking** caused by filamentous bacteria (like *Sphaerotilus natans*) can cause local pollution; this method removes **75-95% of the BOD**
    - ❖ **Trickling filters**: other commonly used method; **sewage** sprayed over rocks or molded plastic; a biofilm of aerobic microbes grows on the rock or plastic; with air circulating throughout rock bed, the aerobic microbes in the slime layer can oxidize much of the organic material "trickling" over the surfaces into carbon dioxide and water; this method removes **80-85% of the BOD**
    - ❖ **Rotating biological contactor***:* another biofilm-based design; consists of **disks** which rotate in water; rotation provides aeration and contact between the biofilm and waste water
- **Disinfection and Release**
  - ✓ Treated sewage is disinfected, usually by chlorination, before discharged; discharged usually into an ocean or flowing streams
- **Sludge Digestion**
  - ✓ **Sludge** can accumulate in: primary sedimentation tanks, activated and trickling secondary treatments
  - ✓ For further treatment, sludge pumped into **anaerobic sludge digesters**
  - ✓ **These digesters** degrade organic matter to produce simpler organic compounds, methane, and carbon dioxide
  - ✓ Three stages in **sludge digestion**
    - ❖ Production of carbon dioxide and organic acids from **anaerobic fermentation**
    - ❖ The organic acids metabolized to form hydrogen and carbon dioxide, as well as organic acids (like acetic acid)
    - ❖ The hydrogen, carbon dioxide, and organic acid (like acetic) are used by methane-producing bacteria to produce methane
  - ✓ **Excess sludge** can be removed, dried, and disposed of, or incinerated
- **Septic Tanks**
  - ✓ In areas of low population density, not connected to municipal sewage systems use **septic tanks**
  - ✓ **Sewage** enters a holding tank; suspended material settles out**; sludge** is pumped out of septic tank periodically and disposed of; the **effluent** flows through a perforated

system of pipes, into a leaching field, where it enters the soil and is decomposed by soil microbes

- **Oxidation Ponds**
  - ✓ Used by many small communities and industries for water treatment; also called **lagoons** or **stabilization ponds**
  - ✓ Inexpensive; require large areas of land
  - ✓ First stage: similar to **primary sewage treatment**
  - ✓ Second stage: roughly similar to **secondary treatment;** effluent is pumped into adjoining pond (s) which are shallow enough to be aerated by wave motion; algae growth encouraged to produce oxygen
  - ✓ Places like campgrounds, highway rest stops use an **oxidative ditch** for **sewage treatment**
- <u>**Tertiary Sewage Treatment**</u>
  - ✓ Developed in some communities; an additional treatment
  - ✓ Designed to remove essentially all the **BOD,** nitrogen, and phosphorus from water
  - ✓ System makes use of **physical filtration and chemical treatments**, rather than biological treatment
  - ✓ Provides drinkable water, but process is very expensive

MICROBIOLOGY

APPLIED AND INDUSTRIAL MICROBIOLOGY

A. Food Microbiology
- Many of the earliest methods of preserving food (heating, cooling, drying, adding sugars and salts, fermentation) still used today
- **Foods and Diseases**
  - Communities have set up local agencies which inspect dairies and restaurants, to minimize the potential of disease outbreaks
  - **Hazard Analysis and Critical Control Point (HACCP) system:** intended to safeguard food from "the farm to the table"; prevent means of contamination
- **Industrial Food Canning**
  - Tries to use the minimum amount of heat necessary to prevent spoilage by organisms, such as *Clostridium botulinum*, without affecting appearance or taste
  - Industrial food canning undergoes "**commercial sterilization**" by steam under pressure in a **retort**
  - Process (1) washing, sorting, blanching→(2) filling can→(3)steaming→(4) can sealed→[**retort:** (5) sterilization by pressurized steam]→(6) cooling→(7) labeling/storing
  - **Commercial sterilization** intends to kill *Clostridium botulinum* endospores
  - Heat is applied for the 12D treatment (12-decimal reductions)
  - **Certain thermophilic endospore-forming bacteria** are resistant to heat treatment; these bacteria are obligate thermophiles and usually remain dormant at temperatures **lower** 45°C (113°F), and are not considered a spoilage problem
    - **Spoilage of Canned Food:** occurs when thermophilics (often anaerobic in low-acid canned foods) exposed to high temperatures; called **thermophilic anaerobic spoilage: cans swell** from the gas; contents have a lowered pH; can be caused by thermophilic species of *Clostridium*; if **thermophilic spoilage** occurs, but **no swelling** of can, called **flat sour spoilage**, caused by organisms such as *Geobacillus stearothermophilus*; **mesophilic bacteria** spoils canned food if food is under processed or leakage of can occurs; certain acidic foods (tomatoes) are preserved by processing temperatures of 100°C or below (will kill: molds, yeasts, certain vegetative bacteria); there are a few microbes which are heat-resistant acid-tolerant microbes: the mold: *Byssochlamys fulva, Aspergillus*; bacterium: *Bacillus coagulans*
- **Aseptic Packaging**
  - Process where "**packages**" are made of material which cannot tolerate conventional heat treatment
  - The **packaging material** can come in rolls, which are fed into a machine which sterilize material with **hot hydrogen peroxide,** sometimes with the aid of UV light then
  - While still in the sterile environment, material is formed into "**packages**" and then filled with liquid food; example: Hi-C
  - Metal containers can be sterilized by: superheated steam, high temperature methods, high electron beams
- **Radiation and Industrial Food Preservation**
  - Works by inhibiting DNA synthesis and prevents reproduction in microbes, insect, plants
  - X rays, gamma rays, high energy accelerators

- o Dosage of radiation needed to kill come in various ranges: low doses (kills insects), pasteurizing doses (on meats and poultry to elimate certain microbes), high doses (to sterilize or lower bacterial populations)
- o Used for foods eaten by: military, astronauts, immunocompromised patients; also used for medical devices
- o Taste of food altered
- **High Pressure Food Preservation**
  - o Used on prewrapped foods (fruits, deli meats, precooked chicken strips)
  - o Items submerged into tanks of pressurized water; process kills many bacteria by disrupting many cellular functions
  - o Preserves color and taste of foods
- **The Role of Microorganisms in Food Processing**
  - o Understanding the relationships between specific microbes and their production of common foods
    - **Cheese: all** require the making of **curd** [(the solid portion separated from the liquid (**whey**)]; **curd** is made up of a protein **casein,** usually formed by the enzymatic action of **rennin** (or **chymosin**), which is helped by certain lactic acid-producing bacteria
    - The lactic acid bacteria also provide different flavors and aromas
    - **Curd** undergoes a "ripening" process; the longer the incubation time, the higher the acidity and sharpness in taste
    - Hard cheese*:* anaerobic bacteria (example: *Propionibacterium*) grow on the interior
    - Semisoft cheese*:* bacteria grow on the surface; *Penicillium*
    - Soft cheese*: Penicillium* grows on the surface
  - o **Other Dairy Products**
    - **Butter:** made by churning cream until fat globules of butter separate from the liquid buttermilk
    - **Buttermilk:** commercially made by inoculating skim milk with bacteria that form lactic acid and diacetyls
    - **Cultured sour cream:** made from cream inoculated with microbes
    - **Yogurt:** commercial yogurt is made from milk in which most of the water has evaporated, and the thickened milk is inoculated with *Streptococcus thermophilus* (acid production) and *Lactobacillus bulgaricus* (flavor and aroma) for several hours
    - **Kefir and kumiss:** both fermented milk beverages (use lactic acid producing bacteria and a lactose-fermenting yeast)
  - o **Nondairy Fermentations**
    - Microbes also used in baking
    - **Breads:** sugars in bread dough fermented by yeasts (*Saccharomyces cervisiae*)
    - **Sauerkraut, pickles, olives:** also undergo the process of fermentation
    - **Soy sauce:** produced by molds (*Aspergillus*)
  - o **Alcoholic Beverages and Vinegar**
    - Almost all alcoholic beverages are produced by microorganisms
    - **Beer and ale:** products of grain starches (example: barley) fermented by yeast; **malting** is the process of converting **raw grain into glucose and maltose**; **malt:** the germinated barley grains contain **maltose, glucose**, and **amylase**; the sugars can then be fermented by yeast, into ethanol and carbon dioxide
    - **Sake:** Japanese rice wine; made with rice without malting; mold *Aspergillus* is first used to convert rice's starch to sugars that can be fermented
    - **Distilled spirits** (whiskey, vodka, rum): carbohydrates from potatoes, cereal grains, molasses are fermented to alcohol; alcohol distilled to make a concentrated alcoholic beverage

- **Wines:** made from fruits; fruits contain sugars that yeasts can directly ferment; malting not necessary; **lactic acid bacteria** convert **malic acid** to the weaker **lactic acid,** a process called **malolactic fermentation;** result is a less acidic, better tasting wine
  - **Vinegar:** is **wine** in which bacteria (*Acetobacter* and *Gluconobacter*) convert the **ethanol into acetic acid;** first, anaerobic fermentation of carbohydrates, by yeast; next the ethanol aerobically oxidized to acetic acid

B. Industrial Microbiology

- Has advanced due to genetically modified organisms using **recombinant DNA technology,** now called **biotechnology**
- **Fermentation Technology**
  - **Industrial Fermentation:** is the cultivation of large amounts of microbes, single cells, plants, animals, to produce **a commercial product** (monoclonal antibodies, insulin, GH)
  - **Bioreactor:** the vessels used in **industrial fermentation;** designed with close attention to **aeration, pH, temperature;** the "continuously stirring type" is the most widely used design; the harvested product, at completion of the fermentation, is known as **batch production**
  - The **microbes** in **industrial fermentation** produce **two** types of **metabolites:**
    - **Primary metabolite** (example: product ethanol): the **primary metabolite** is formed as the cell grows **(growth/trophophase) stage;** the production curve follows the cell population curve almost in parallel, with minimal lag
    - **Secondary metabolites** (example: penicillin): product produced only after the logarithmic **growth (trophophase) phase** of the cell is completed; the main production occurs during the **stationary phase (idiophase)**
  - **Strain improvement** also a continuous process in industrial microbiology; a **strain** differs physiologically; it may have an enzyme which carries out a particular activity or lacks such an activity; in producing **mutant strains (**via UV, X rays, nitrogen mustards**),** one is able to increase production of a desired product (example: Penicillium)
- **Immobilized Enzymes and Microorganisms**
  - Many industries are using **free enzymes** isolated from microbes to manufacture products, such as paper, textiles, syrups
  - These **enzymes do not** produce costly or toxic waste products and work under safe, moderate conditions
  - Most of these **enzymes** are **immobilized** (attached to spheres or fibers), so they can convert a continuous flow of **substrate to product,** without being lost
- **Industrial Products**
  - Microbiologists are devising alternative uses for old products and creating new ones
    - **Amino Acids: glutamic acid** (used to make flavor enhancer monosodium glutamate (MSG)); **lysine** and **methionine** (synthesized as cereal food supplements); **phenylalanine** and **aspartic acid** (sweeteners)
    - **Citric Acid:** component of citrus fruits; a product of **mold metabolism** (*Aspergillus niger*); (antioxidant, tartness and flavor to food, pH adjuster)
    - **Enzymes: amylases** (made by mold *Aspergillus*, produce syrup from cornstarch, paper sizing, production of glucose from starch); **proteases** (make breads, meat tenderizers, detergents); **glucose isomerase** (sweetener)**; rennin** (form curds in milk, cheese production)
    - **Vitamins:** used as food supplements; **Vitamin B12** (*Psedomonas, Propionibacterium* species); **Vitamins B2** (fungi *Ashbya gossypiiand*); **Vitamin C** (*Acetobacter*)
    - **Pharmaceuticals:** use to make **antibiotics** (*Streptomyces hygroscopius*), **vaccine, steroids** (cortisone, estrogens, progesterone)
    - **Copper Extraction by Leaching:** the bacteria *Thiobacillus ferroxidans* helps recover **copper ore**

- ▪ **Microorganisms as Industrial Products: baker's yeast** (for home baking); mixture of *Rhizobium* and *Bradyrhizobium* with **peat moss** ensures moisture; *Bacillus thuringiensis* is an insect **pathogen** (control leaf-eating insect larvae)
- ● **Alternative Energy Sources Using Microorganisms**
  - ○ With diminished supplies and increasing cost of **fossil fuels, renewable energy resources** will increase
  - ○ One **energy source** is **biomass**: collective **organic matter**, produced by living organisms; microbes can be used to convert **biomass** into **"alternative energy"** through a process called **bioconversion**
  - ○ **Methane:** one of the most convenient energy sources produced from **bioconversion**
  - ○ **Methane:** produced from wastes in landfill sites, and can be used for energy
- ● **Biofuels**
  - ○ **Biofuels:** renewable replacement fuels
  - ○ Includes **alcohol (ethanol:** mainly from corn, sugarcane**), hydrogen** (from microbial fermentation), **oils** (from algae)
- ● **Industrial Microbiology and the Future**

Microbes will always remain an important part of many basic food-processing technologies; **genetic engineering** has expanded the potential for new products

Printed in the United States
By Bookmasters